THE GOD EFFECT

HOW SUGGESTION AND RITUAL SHAPE RELIGION AND MEDICINE THROUGH PLACEBO RESPONSES

Colin Brewer

Foreword by
Edzard Ernst

SOCIETAS
essays in political
& cultural criticism

imprint-academic.com

Published in the UK by
Imprint Academic Ltd., PO Box 200, Exeter EX5 5YX, UK

Distributed in the USA by
Lightning Source,
La Vergne, TN 37086, USA

ISBN 9781788361439 paperback

A CIP catalogue record for this book is available from the
British Library and US Library of Congress

This product complies with the General Product Safety Regulations
introduced by the European Union in 2024.

EU GPSR Authorised Representative:
LOGOS EUROPE, 9 rue Nicolas Poussin,
17000, LA ROCHELLE, France

E-mail: Contact@logoseurope.eu

sets up so that we can all face our belief-systems, whether theist or atheist, with a heightened self-scrutiny and transparency. I share his positivity regarding ritual and its ability to explore the deeper truths of the human self and, what Larkin termed, 'the million petalled flower of being here'. I also agree with many of his criticisms of religion when it is inhumane and when a defensive certainty takes the oxygen out of the air. Whilst I remain of the mind that ultimately reality is worthy of our trust, I find more to engage honestly with here in this book than I do with many religious fundamentalists or the casually indifferent." — *Mark Oakley, Dean of Southwark*

"An original and thought-provoking exploration of the parallels between placebo effects and religious belief, written with clarity and clinical insight. A stimulating contribution to public understanding of medicine, religion and secularism." — *Keith Porteous Wood, President, (UK) National Secular Society*

By the same author

Can social work survive?

Antabuse treatment for alcoholism

Medical management of alcohol and opiate abuse (Editor

I'll see myself out, thank you (Editor)

Let me not get Alzheimer's, sweet heaven!

Contents

Preface

When I began writing what eventually became this book about placebo effects and religion, I reflected that I might also, coincidentally, be writing the longest suicide note in history. In the early 2000s, I experienced several extremely stressful years when six colleagues and I were awaiting a hearing by the General Medical Council following complaints about treatments at the addiction clinic I had established in the 1980s. With one exception, the complaints came not from patients or their families but mainly from members of the British addiction 'establishment', some of whom had previously been forced to apologise to us very publicly. The exception, added only very late in the day to the other charges, involved the death of one of our patients.[1] It all weighed very heavily on me, as did the feeling of responsibility for the involvement of my colleagues in the proceedings. It is very common for physicians to feel suicidal in this situation and an alarming number do actually take their own lives. I came very close to doing so, partly because I thought that my suicide might make the proceedings easier for my colleagues and attempts by doctors rarely fail. Thinking that if I did go the whole way, I should leave some sort of personal and professional memoir, I started writing and it turned out to be quite therapeutic. As well as many case histories (which feature in a forthcoming book about addiction treatment) it included reflections on the prescribing of placebos, common when I qualified but supposedly abandoned and unethical by the millennium. A few years after my erasure from the medical register, I returned to the memoir and expanded its scope to include the many similarities between placebo effects in religious procedures and the procedures of both conventional and 'alternative' medicine. People often feel much better after injections or tablets that contain no active or pharmacologically useful substances. In the same way, they often feel much better after prayers or pilgrimages addressed to a god who, many British and West European citizens seem to have concluded, does not exist or, like Einstein, Voltaire, Hume, Spinoza and many other leading thinkers, that if He does exist, He does not care.

Religion has always interested me though mainly in an anthropological way and when I started my psychiatric career, I incorporated that interest into the therapeutically important doctor-patient relationship. As well as routinely asking patients 'What is your religion?' I always asked how important religion was in their lives, because that could influence the management of their problems. When one patient cancelled an appointment at the last minute, I spent the next hour tabulating the responses in about a hundred case-notes. Only about 12% of my mostly well-educated, White British private patients had said that religion was important to them. Some of those added that they adhered to no particular faith but firmly believed in some sort of god or were 'very spiritual'.

On my first day at St. Bartholomew's Hospital medical school, the Dean, an Evangelical Christian who helped to found the Christian Medical Fellowship, told the new student intake, which included a few Muslims, Hindus and Buddhists as well as unbelievers, that we could not be good doctors unless we were good Christians. Several fellow-students planned to become missionaries. Fortunately, during most of my adolescence I had experienced a less fundamentalist and cocksure version of Christianity at a school run by Quakers, probably the least doctrinaire of all religious sects. There were no sermons and if you disagreed with what someone said during a Quaker meeting, you could say so. The school also introduced me to J S Bach's great choral works, which I later sang in some of Europe's great cathedrals. Quakers were often non-committal about God and the Trinity but nevertheless seemed keener than most people on doing good deeds. You can only become a Quaker when you have attended several meetings and reached the age of discretion but by that time, despite these good examples, I had come down on the sceptical, evidence-demanding side of the fence. As a medical student, my first letter to a national newspaper (pseudonymous and simplistic but published because a cousin was its foreign correspondent) asked why a supposedly benevolent deity had allowed several hundred people to die when a French dam collapsed. Later, as a medical journalist, I often wrote about the interface – not always congenial - between medicine and doctrinaire religions.

I qualified at a time when the deliberate use of placebos, without telling patients, was regarded as perfectly normal, with results that often pleased both parties. During psychiatric training, my favourite mentor decided to give sham ECT (electro-convulsive treatment) to a depressed patient who had previously had several courses and wanted another. He thought she didn't need the real thing, so without informing her, we gave

2

her the anaesthetic but no electricity and she recovered as quickly as usual. Within a decade, such withholding of information would be regarded as seriously unethical. Something similar but on a much larger scale occurred accidentally at a Midlands psychiatric hospital in 1974. For two years, because of a faulty machine, its ECT patients never received electricity but neither the nurses nor the doctors noticed. In 1980, a formal controlled trial of real vs sham ECT in depression unresponsive to antidepressant drugs showed that real ECT was indeed more effective - but not very much more.

Only in the past few years has research into placebo effects and related phenomena become an academic discipline in its own right, as opposed to studying them as complicating factors in the randomized controlled trials that allow doctors to say with high confidence whether or not a given treatment is truly and specifically effective. Before the 1990s, an equivalent evidence-base for Complementary and Alternative Medicine (CAM) hardly existed until pioneers like Prof Edzard Ernst subjected a wide range of CAM procedures to the same sceptical scrutiny that is now routine in orthodox medical practice. Studies by him and a growing international band of researchers repeatedly found that nearly all CAM treatments were not more effective than comparable sham or placebo procedures, the exceptions being only marginally more effective. However, they also found that placebo and non-specific effects could be surprisingly large in both CAM and conventional medicine. You can draw your own conclusions from the fact that the then Prince Charles, a long-time promotor of CAM, initially welcomed Prof Ernst's appointment but became steadily less welcoming as the negative evidence-base became steadily larger and more incontrovertible. As King Charles, he continues to promote CAM and has appointed another CAM supporter as head of his medical household at Buckingham Palace.

I hope this book gives the general reader an idea of the surprising power of mind over body, as shown by both placebo effects and hypnosis and in both medical and religious settings. It is also a record of a dying generation of British doctors for the benefit of later graduates who missed out on these highly educational experiences. Finally, as I was told by Prof Fabrizio Benedetti, the grandfather of modern placebo research, it is about time that somebody wrote a book about the placebo aspects of religion. As far as I know, this is the first.

Foreword

Colin Brewer's book explores the powerful, often unconscious, influence of the placebo effect across various human experiences. It explains that the perceived benefits from religious practices and many medical treatments, especially those involving Complementary and Alternative Medicine, are not due to inherent efficacy but to factors like expectation, suggestion, faith and conditioning. It examines how rituals, suggestive environments, and charismatic figures in both religion and medicine can trigger positive responses – and sometimes negative ones.

Put simply, the placebo effect is the phenomenon where a patient's health improves after receiving an inert treatment, like a sugar pill or saline injection. The patient improves not because of any action of the medication but because he or she hopes and believes it will work.

For physicians, the placebo is a more or less constant companion throughout their careers. It is always present and comes in many different guises. When I was told at medical school that a doctor who cannot generate a placebo response in his patients should become a pathologist, I was amused. When, as a budding clinician, I noted that my patients often reported symptom relief even after a purely diagnostic intervention, I was puzzled. When I realised that doctors do not need a placebo in order to generate a placebo response – all treatments provoke a placebo response, and all therapeutic outcomes are at least partly due to placebo – I was delighted. When, as a clinical researcher, I needed to differentiate between the specific and the non-specific (placebo) effects of a therapy, the placebo was an irritating distraction. When I had to develop suitable placebos to scientifically test all sorts of alternative therapies ranging from acupuncture to spiritual healing, I was excited to cover new ground. When I encountered the research of neuroscientists on the actions of placebos in the brain, I was fascinated.

Colin Brewer expands this already wide and colourful spectrum of perspectives on placebo by drawing intriguing parallels between the placebo effect and religion. The common denominator, it seems, is what we today often call "mind over matter". The responses of both placebo and religion are based on belief, suggestion, hope and expectation and possibly also conditioning.

The ritual of the medical consultation, the trust in the doctor, the past experiences, and the physical act of administering a therapy all contribute to this powerful belief, which then triggers reactions within our body.

Similarly, religion can leverage belief, hope and expectation to produce profound effects on the believer. The "mind over matter" aspect in this context is a mechanism for psychological, emotional, and even physical well-being. Just like medical rituals, religious rituals—such as prayer, pilgrimage, meditation, or specific ceremonies—can create a conditioned response. Over time, these practices become associated with feelings of comfort, and well-being.

In essence, the "mind over matter" phenomenon common to both the placebo effect and religion reflects our brain's ability to employ belief – whether in a pill, a person, a ritual, or a god (any god) - to influence the body's internal state and the attitude of patients to their symptoms, especially pain. It's a testament to the powerful connection between our psychological world and our physiological reality.

As Humanists, we find the basis for morality in the concern for the well-being of others. We aim to treat others as we would like to be treated ourselves. This book is also a celebration of Humanism. Colin Brewer empathetically shines light on a variety of "mind over matter" phenomena from a whole range of different perspectives. He avoids jargon and his writing is entertaining as well as informative. This book, the first of its kind, deserves to be read by a wide audience and I hope you find it as inspiring as I did.

Edzard Ernst
Cambridge
September 2025

Chapter 1
Introduction

Go, go, go, said the bird: human kind
Cannot bear very much reality.
Time past and time future
What might have been and what has been
Point to one end, which is always present.
T.S. Eliot. Burnt Norton.

It is good to know the truth but it is better to be happy.
Russian proverb.

We all believe what makes life easier to bear.
Steven Vizinczey. If Only.

When we are asked to choose between truth and contentment, most of us
pick contentment.
Christopher Hedges. War is a force that gives us meaning.

A well-educated American woman with irritable bowel syndrome
feels much better after a course of acupuncture; but the acupuncturist
has used a special, deceptive non-needle that never penetrated her skin.
After being shown a Latin text supposedly from the Bible, a woman
accused of witchcraft writhes and curses, regarded in Renaissance
France as a sure sign that she is possessed by demons; but the Latin text
is actually from a poem by Virgil. In 2004, the Iraqi government pays
large sums for bomb-detecting devices that cost a few cents to build and
do not detect bombs; but the government insists that they are effective.
A prosperous Libyan merchant, who believes that his aches and pains are
due to a snake that has somehow entered his stomach, is cured when a
surgeon operates and shows him, after he emerges from anaesthesia, the
small snake that he has removed; but the incision is only superficial
(though impressively sutured and dressed) and the snake had been
captured beforehand. In 1870, two young men recover from severe
bacterial pneumonia. One attributes his recovery to medicines that have
no pharmacological curative effects. The other attributes it to Latin
prayers that have no heavenly curative effects and to holy relics of a 14th
century saint that may not have really come from the saint's body.

This book is about the threads that link these very diverse scenarios.
In medical contexts they are mainly known as placebo and non-specific
effects and until about forty years ago, they were largely ignored,
dismissed as trivial and transient or regarded as undesirable noise in the
system. Noise that made it difficult to interpret the randomized
controlled trials of treatment, now correctly called 'evidence-based

medicine', that progressively freed medicine and surgery, though not 'complementary and alternative medicine' (CAM), from drugs and procedures that at best had no specific effects and at worst made sick patients even sicker. When religious beliefs and rituals are aimed at relieving physical or mental distress, the many similarities with placebo and non-specific effects have rarely been recognized or recorded, even though once pointed out, they are – as you will soon discover – rather obvious. They are particularly obvious to doctors of my generation, who were the last of several millennia of physicians for whom the deliberate prescribing of placebos was a daily and therapeutically important feature of medical practice. That lack of recognition may have something to do with the fact that until the late 19th century in Britain, to suggest that the god of prayers, pilgrimages and holy relics did not exist or did not care could seriously damage one's professional and social life and even one's liberty. Fortunately, the total absence of direct evidence for the existence of the Judaeo-Christian-Muslim god, like the similar total absence of evidence where most of 'alternative' medicine is concerned, does not mean that prayer, pilgrimage and relics have no benefits. It is just that the benefits do not require the existence of the god, just as the benefits of placebo tablets and injections do not require the existence of any disease-modifying pharmacological activity.

A few more examples. A Belgian surgeon is able to do delicate operations on the thyroid gland with less bleeding than usual; but the patients have received neither local nor general anaesthetics. A government introduces a policy that it claims will reduce crime, suicide or unemployment. Reductions may actually occur but are entirely due to factors other than the new policies. A teenaged patient with severe icthyosis ('fish skin'), an incurable, genetically-determined congenital skin disease, often fatal in childhood, is not helped even by repeated skin grafts from unaffected areas; but to everyone's surprise, he improves considerably following hypnosis, one limb at a time. Rabbits fed a cholesterol-rich diet develop arteriosclerosis; but if they have been held and petted several times a day, the changes are only half as severe compared with an unpetted control group.

Placebo and non-specific effects can be extremely powerful and I will argue that doctors and other health professionals should learn how to make better use of them but they are not limited to patients with painful or life-altering conditions. The same conscious and unconscious psychological mechanisms that can relieve pain and despair and improve function are also involved in aspects of life ranging from prayers, pilgrimages and the creation of saints to Olympic athletics, politics, war, gastronomy and the prison sentences imposed by judges. In particular, placebo and non-specific effects partly explain the origins of religion and completely explain the beneficial effects of religious rituals designed to relieve spiritual, emotional and physical pain. Unlike the 'new atheists' (actually less unkind and abrasive than their Victorian forebears) my main aim is not to bring about the disappearance of religious beliefs, an extremely unlikely outcome even in an increasingly secular Western Europe. Instead, it is to help both religious and non-religious people to see religion's everyday rituals and beliefs in a new but still positive light; and perhaps to reduce the number of people who are influenced by the intolerant, anti-rational and historically unsound or absurd facets of religion. Those facets are raising the spectre of a new Holy Inquisition, blasphemy laws and even of modern wars of religion in Europe when we thought they had largely disappeared in 1648 after the Peace of Westphalia ended the frightful slaughter of the Thirty Years War between Protestants and Roman Catholics.

For thousands of years, shamans, priests and physicians helped many sick people to feel better. They believed they could cure them of life-threatening diseases as well as less serious ones but most of that relief and recovery had nothing to do with the medication that was prescribed, the gods that were worshipped or the specific features of healing and religious rituals. Until barely a century ago, physicians were mainly walking and talking (and listening) placebos but they still had useful and important functions and considerable prestige. To help us understand why so many people came to have so much faith in religion and medicine, let us go just a little further back in history by imagining two scenarios, both set in about 1870. Anaesthesia and anti-bacterial surgical techniques have recently been introduced. Doctors, as a profession, feel increasingly effective and important and Joseph Lister will soon be knighted by Queen Victoria for making surgery very much safer. Later, he will become the first medical member of the House of Lords.

In the first scenario, Gerald, a 20-year-old with a bad cough and a high fever, feels very ill. He is terrified that he might die because his younger brother succumbed to a similar condition a couple of years earlier when travelling abroad. Every breath is painful. The cause of the fever and the pain is lobar pneumonia due to a common bacterium, pneumococcus, though the existence and importance of bacteria are only just beginning to be recognised and they have not yet been classified. (The dyes so essential for distinguishing between different bacteria under the microscope are only just being discovered or synthesised.) Household remedies do nothing for the fever, which is, in any case, a normal and, up to a point, helpful component of the body's mechanisms for combating infections. Fortunately, the generous amount of opium in Dr J Collis Browne's popular Chlorodyne Mixture, purchasable, like opium pills, without a prescription at any pharmacy, eases the pain and helps Gerald to sleep, but the fever gets worse. His family are prosperous and modern-minded and they summon Sir Bentley Foxton, a prominent, modern-minded doctor who is also one of Queen Victoria's physicians, hence his knighthood. He is a tall, impressive man and after a thorough and unhurried physical examination, he prescribes several medicines. He also reassures Gerald that he will recover. Gerald immediately feels a little better and less feverish, though a thermometer would have shown no reduction in his temperature. He feels better still after the first doses of the medicines. Two days later, the fever settles and after a week, he is out of bed and clearly on the mend. His family happily pay Sir Bentley's fees and their wine merchant sends him several cases of champagne for good measure.

In the second scenario, Henri, also 20 years old but living in Étrépigny, a small French village, has the same condition, the same symptoms and similar fears about dying. He too has lost a brother to pneumonia. His family have given him a popular local folk remedy made from plants with healing reputations but it did not help. They are not prosperous and there is no doctor nearer than Charleville-Mézières 20 kilometres away but they have great faith in God and they summon the village priest, to whose sermons they listen respectfully every Sunday. When he arrives, he makes reassuring prognostications, then kneels and confidently intones a prayer for Henri's recovery. It is in Latin, which Henri, though literate, doesn't really understand but associates with wisdom, learning and God. It makes him feel that he is benefiting from direct access to the deity. The priest finishes by laying his hands on Henri's head before pressing a small gold and glass reliquary, containing a visible fragment of bone, onto the area of Henri's chest that hurts so much when he breathes. Immediately, Henri feels less pain, less feverish and more hopeful. Morning and evening, he recites a special prayer in French that the priest has written down for him. In a couple of days, the fever and pain abate and in a week or so, Henri too is able to rise from his bed, still weak but improving by the day.

Since I control this narrative, I know, from my 21st century vantage point, that nothing prescribed for Gerald by Sir Bentley could have had any significant pharmacological effect on the pneumococcal lung infection that caused his pain and fever. I know this because I know what drugs were available to doctors in the 1860s and I know that there is no evidence that any of them kills bacteria in the lungs or stimulates the body's natural defences. Spontaneous, rapid and complete recovery from lobar pneumonia, with or without treatment, was common in healthy young men and that is what happened here. It accounts for the fall in temperature after a few days and the subsequent steady recovery. If Gerald felt better after Sir Bentley's visit and the first dose of medicine, that was because he shared a general but unfounded belief that doctors knew a lot about the causes of illness and that their medicines were often effective. That explains the immediate improvement in pain and anxiety. Gerald wanted and expected to feel better and his mind obliged by bending his perceptions in the required direction. What I have described are some of the basic placebo and non-specific effects that mediate and often powerfully reinforce all pharmacological, psychological and surgical interventions, whether or not the interventions have any real and specific effects on the disease process.

As to Henri, my explanation is not very different. Theists, especially monotheists, who firmly believe in a deity who responds promptly and effectively to all prayers for healing may not agree but like Einstein, a large minority or more of educated citizens in most Western European countries reject the idea of a concerned deity. ("I cannot imagine a God who rewards and punishes the objects of his creation, whose purposes are modelled after our own; a God, in short, who is but a reflection of human frailty. Neither can I believe that the individual survives the death of his body, although feeble souls harbour such thoughts through fear or ridiculous egotisms.")[2] Alternatively, they have serious doubts about His existence or simply think that the hypothesis is so unconvincing as to be not worth bothering about. All of them will probably agree that Henri's recovery was not a result of divine intervention; had nothing to do with Latin or French prayers or the application of holy relics; and was due to entirely natural bodily processes and defence mechanisms, without which human and animal life would be impossible. Indeed, as we shall see in Chapter 3, the Étrépigny priest may not even believe in the Christian god. The fact that like Gerald, Henri began to feel better and more hopeful as soon as the visiting professional began his ministrations and continued to feel better even before the fever broke was mainly a manifestation of the placebo and non-specific effects of religion, including impressive rituals and the effects of authoritative and persuasive reassurance almost regardless of the nature of that authority. In both cases, the improvement in morale caused by faith in the visitor's professional abilities and beliefs, as well as by physical contact with him, might have boosted the body's immune system in ways that could be helpful in pneumonia but harmful in other conditions but those changes reflect the *intensity* of faith, not its object. Intense faith in Krishna, Mohammed, Zeus, Thor or the superiority of Soviet medicine would have had similar effects.

Though these case-histories are imaginary, they are not at all unimaginable but it might be thought unfair to use spontaneous recovery from a short-lived illness to illustrate placebo and non-specific effects. Let us look at a real case history that shows how those effects relieved a distressing condition that had been present for some time and had resisted treatment. In the 1920s, Alberto di Pirajno was an Italian doctor working in Libya when it was still divided into the Italian colonies of Cyrenaica and Tripolitania. His delightful memoir is called 'A cure for serpents'[3] and the case that provides the title was that of a leading citizen, "the rich but munificent Hajj Ahmed es-Sed", who became convinced that a serpent had entered his mouth and stomach while he slept in the open. Whether the abdominal pain of which he complained was a pre-existing condition made worse by the supposed serpent or whether it was an understandable consequence of the belief is not made clear but it had resisted all the traditional remedies, both pharmacological and amuletical. Worse, his father had appeared to him in a dream and confirmed the presence and malevolence of the serpent. Di Pirajno thought that Hajj Ahmed was "in the period of the male menopause" and not adapting well to ageing but attempts to persuade him that his stomach was snake-free were unsuccessful.

One day, Hajj Ahmed asked di Pirajno if he could operate on him to remove the snake. Di Pirajno eventually, and very reluctantly, agreed but what he actually did was not quite what Hajj Ahmed requested. Under general anaesthesia, Pirajno made a very superficial abdominal incision only a millimetre or two deep into the skin over the stomach but long enough, as he reports, "for the extraction of even a young crocodile", following which he stitched it up and his assistant "executed a most artistic bandage". When the patient awoke, he was shown a small snake that had been specially captured for the purpose. Pirajno reports that after this procedure, the pains disappeared. He also writes that he felt unhappy that Hajj Ahmed's importunities persuaded him "to cross the narrow line that separates the physician from the charlatan" but I think he is being too self-critical. To me, a charlatan is someone who, for entirely commercial reasons, actively encourages people to use a medicine or procedure that he knows to have no specific effect and who often promotes that particular intervention to the exclusion of others. For healers who sincerely believe and specialise in treatments that mostly lack good evidence of specific effects, some other term than 'charlatan' is needed. 'Practitioners of Complementary and Alternative Medicine' (CAM)[4] will do for the moment but di Pirajno was a conventional salaried, colonial doctor, like his British Empire equivalents. All the encouragement to operate came from his patient. The great Renaissance Humanist writer Montaigne described a patient very like Hajj Ahmed, except that she believed her throat pains were due to an inadvertently swallowed needle. The doctors could find no needle but the pain continued until they gave her an emetic and "secretly placed a needle in the vomitus".[5]

You would be wrong to think that the health-beliefs of unsophisticated early-20th century Libyans or 16th century French housewives must be far removed from the health-beliefs of educated citizens of first-world countries in the 21st century. In reality, while some ancient imagined causes of disease have receded, others have simply been revised and several new ones have appeared. In the West, spirit or diabolic possessions are much rarer than they were in 17th century England and North America but the Roman Catholic church is only one among several religions that will provide an exorcism on request; and belief in spirit possession and witchcraft is still very prominent in many less sophisticated communities. For alleged serpents in the stomach causing pain and illness, substitute any number of alleged allergies, vitamin and mineral deficiencies, unspecified 'toxins', emanations from electricity cables or supposed infections with mysterious but maddeningly elusive viruses.

If many doctors today have little awareness of just how extremely powerful placebo effects can be, that is mainly because unlike the steadily diminishing survivors of my generation of physicians, they have been strongly discouraged from using placebos deliberately because that usually involves deception; and since the 1970s, deceiving patients, even for their benefit, has been increasingly regarded by the professional bodies in most developed countries as unethical.[6] I qualified in 1963 during what was, in retrospect, the autumn of placebo medicines. Even then, not many doctors regarded placebo and non-specific effects (terms that will soon get considerable expansion) with the seriousness, the respect and, at times, the jaw-dropping amazement that they deserve because the double-blind Randomised Controlled Trials (RCTs) that demonstrate and quantify those effects were only just beginning to become routine. The best RCTs compare the treatment in question with an appropriate placebo or with another treatment that has previously proved superior to a placebo. To minimise bias for or against, they are also double-blind, i.e. neither patients nor the assessing clinicians know to which group an individual patient has been allocated until the trial is over. Until very recently, placebo effects were seen mainly as undesirable noise in the system that got in the way of interpreting clinical trials. They were not often studied as interesting and important phenomena in themselves. Even more rarely were they studied with a view to maximising them or even analysing them in individual patients. Doctors who deliberately treated patients with placebos, as some still do, rarely published their experiences. It is only in retirement that I feel able to publish mine outside of medical journals but unlike many medical writers who dismiss or belittle placebo and non-specific effects, I shall argue that precisely because they can be so powerful, we should explore ways of using them in an ethical way for the benefit of our patients.

Good Randomised Controlled Trials are crucially important and form the main evidence-base both for the specific effectiveness of most of today's treatments and for the ineffectiveness of many others that led to their abandonment by modern medicine. However, just as important as RCTs is one of the broadly philosophical principles that define and inform them: the null hypothesis. In medicine, what that boils down to is a *presumption of ineffectiveness*. If there is no evidence from good and preferably repeated RCTs that a particular treatment is more effective than a comparable placebo, then there should be *a presumption that it is not more effective*. That is because even now, many apparently good ideas in medicine turn out to be unhelpful in practice. Very few of those 'breakthroughs' that are publicised almost weekly in the media merit the description. Given this background, it is customary and reasonable for medical scientists to assume that *claims for effectiveness are invalid until otherwise proved*. That's the 'null' part of the null hypothesis. The other part is the principle that it's the duty of the people making such claims to produce the evidence that may disprove the null hypothesis. It is emphatically not the duty of medical science to accept claims of effectiveness simply because somebody asserts them, however persuasive the claims may seem, however desperate the suffering patients and their doctors may feel and however distinguished the claimant. Even if (indeed, *especially* if) King Charles or leading footballers, actors, clothes designers, 'influencers' and TV personalities support them. For medical scientists, the null hypothesis – that the claim is *not* true – is, or should be, a normal part of life. For religions and CAM, it is the hypothesis that dare not speak its name.

The first encounters with placebo and non-specific effects happen very early in our lives. We bruise a knee, get nipped by the family dog or touch something hot. The skin is unbroken but oh, it hurts! Mummy stops what she is doing and hurries to our side and if a simple cuddle and a few soothing words don't do the trick, she offers to kiss it better. In the remote valleys of New Guinea, some other response may be customary but the principle and the effect will be the same. If the injury is minor and the pain transient, the crying will soon stop anyway but even if it less trivial, the kiss often stops the tears or even changes them to a hesitant smile. No PhD-hungry child psychologist has compared kissing it better to other methods of pain relief for minor injuries but I doubt whether any of them would prove more effective.

As our infant vocabulary and concepts expand, additional pain-relieving techniques may be employed. The pain may be shared with a toy, for example, but both mummy and you soon discover that not all toys have the same pain-relieving effect. If you own two teddy-bears, only one of them may work and in this respect you already share some interesting characteristics with Samuel Pepys, who in 1664 wasn't sure whether to attribute his improved health in the previous few months to "my hare's foote, or taking every morning of a pill of turpentine, or my having left off the wearing of a gowne".[7] His health worsened again but a few months later, that indefatigable and priapic diarist was told by his colleague Sir William Batten, who shared his faith in the prophylactic qualities of hare's feet, that Pepys's charm was the wrong sort, because it should include the first joint of the hare's foot and Pepys's didn't. Batten allowed Pepys to hold his own, more potent version for a while and Pepys's response to the new charm is worth quoting in full: "[I]t is a strange thing how fancy works, for I no sooner almost handled his foote but my belly began to be loose and to break wind, and whereas I was in some pain yesterday and t'other day and in fear of more to-day, I became very well, and so continue."[8] He immediately bought a hare for his dinner and made himself a proper charm. Three months later on the 26th of March 1665, he wrote of "...my Hare's-foot, which is my preservative against wind, for I never had a fit of the Collique since I wore it". We can already see that not all placebos are equal and that placebo effects, though universal, are also a very personal thing.

Mummy may suggest soothing the pain with an ointment. That too might bring instant relief but it can't be due to any of the drugs it contains because no drug penetrates unbroken skin that quickly. As with the teddy-bears, you may soon develop a preference for ointment A over ointment B but that will probably owe more to their different smells than to the different chemicals they contain. If she gives you a paediatric pain-killer such as paracetamol, its placebo effects may be more important in relieving pain than paracetamol's very modest pharmacological effects.

When you are older, and if you have a more serious injury or illness, mummy may add her preferred deity to the therapeutic menu by praying to Him, or by encouraging you to pray. He will soon be your preferred deity too. The belief that God takes a personal interest in your welfare and can cure or relieve illness often persists into adulthood and that early implantation of belief and prayer, often lasting a lifetime, probably enhances religion's placebo effects. Anthropologists seem to agree that religious beliefs and practices began with the shamans or medicine-men who were and remain a feature of all societies untouched by the modern world that have been studied by fieldwork or archaeology. They also seem to agree that the power and influence of shamans were based at least partly on their ability to prepare seemingly effective remedies from the hundreds of plants in the fields and forests and from minerals and animal products. Shamans might also seek help from ancestors or tribal deities. The physicians who increasingly took over the shamans' therapeutic role well before the time of Hippocrates, also used these remedies. Modern pharmacology and ethnobotany confirm that many of the plants used by shamans and pre-1920 physicians contained interesting and chemically or physically active compounds. Unfortunately, modern pharmacology also confirms that many of them had toxic rather than healing effects. Most of them were not used for conditions in which they might have been genuinely and specifically effective and they were often used in conditions for which they had no useful pharmacological effect at all. Furthermore, even if we now know that they did have potentially useful effects in some conditions, they were often used in doses that were so small as to be ineffective or so large that they had serious side-effects. For example, there is no evidence that mercury ever cured a single case of syphilis but it must have killed numerous patients and badly damaged the health of many others.

The 'placebo' component of 'placebo and non-specific effects' is the bit that can most obviously be regarded as a 'treatment'. That means the effect of things like tablets, capsules, liquid medicines and injections (especially injections) but also ointments, dressings, physiotherapy, special diets, psychotherapy, radiation (e.g. from lasers) and, of course, surgery. Even when the tablet, ointment or injection contain no active ingredients, or none likely to be helpful in a given illness, the surgeon makes only a symbolic cut into the skin and the laser is not switched on. In conventional medical practice and clinical research today, a 'pure' placebo means something given to a patient that the doctor knows to have no pharmacological activity at all. The terms 'impure' or 'active' placebo are used to describe procedures like di Pirajno's superficial incision, or drugs with names or noticeable but therapeutically irrelevant effects that impress the patient but are thought by the doctor to have no specific effect on the disease process. Pure placebos are what active drugs are compared with in most RCTs. Doctors are not now supposed to use 'pure' placebos in everyday practice but many still use another kind of 'impure' placebo when, for example, they prescribe generally harmless vitamin tablets to well-nourished patients who feel unhappy if they leave a consultation without receiving a prescription.

In this book, I have broadened the range of meanings to include currently used medicines and procedures (like spiritual healing and most other forms of CAM including acupuncture) that are *honestly believed* by the healer, whether medically qualified or not, to have specific therapeutic effects that in reality are unsupported or positively disproved by Randomised Controlled Trials against a placebo medicine or procedure that looks or feels like the real thing. Apart from a few vaccines and anti-serums developed around the end of the 19th c. (notably against diphtheria and rabies) there was no RCT-validated evidence base or a valid underlying theory or rationale for almost the whole of conventional pre-1920 medicines. The 19th century Anglo-American physician Oliver Wendell Holmes said: "If we threw the entire pharmacopoeia into the sea, it would be so much the worse for the fishes and so much the better for our patients". He could have made almost the same suggestion about the pre-1920 doctors who prescribed those medicines. My broadened range also includes the procedures used in the more formalized and elaborate sources of spiritual healing called religions, especially when they are used for the relief of physical and psychological illness. Some of these psychological (or mental, or psychiatric, or spiritual) illnesses have largely psychological symptoms, such as depression and anxiety. Others express themselves with physical symptoms such as pain, palpitations, or fatigue. Conversely, even obviously physical illnesses like cancer or arthritis inevitably produce psychological reactions that can profoundly influence the level of suffering and incapacity. These real, non-imaginary and clinically important components are the main arena in which placebo and non-specific effects work their daily wonders.

The 'non-specific' component, often just as important or even more important in terms of overall effect, includes things like consultations, physical examinations, reassurance, endoscopy, x-rays and blood tests; and, very importantly, putting a name and thus a narrative to the patient's problem. (As the novelist Isaac Dinesen wrote, 'All sorrows can be borne if you put them into a story or tell a story about them'.) Some placebo researchers use the terms 'true' and 'perceived' placebo effects instead[9] but if one can speak of 'tradition' in a field of medicine that has only recently begun to attract anything like the level of attention it deserves, I shall stick with the more traditional 'non-specific' usage, which I think is also more easily understood. These non-specific factors and their symbolic meanings can make patients feel much better but they are features of most therapeutic encounters and are thus not 'specific' to the treatment in question. Non-specific effects also include spontaneous improvement or recovery, as with Gerald and Henri, and the related concept of 'regression to the mean', the finding that among a hundred people with, say, high blood pressure or low haemoglobin levels, a significant proportion will return to normal within a few months without treatment. (To avoid too much repetition, 'placebo effects' will often mean non-specific effects as well.)

Unlike the tablet or capsule of a genuinely and specifically effective drug like penicillin or thyroxine, which will do its specific, pharmacologically-determined job just as well whether it is delivered to the bedside in a plain plastic cup or an emerald-studded Fabergé goblet, the *style* in which the non-specific components are delivered can produce very different outcomes. The length and setting of the consultation. The genuine or apparent thoroughness of the examination. The number and nature of the tests. The doctor's comportment, appearance, and tone of voice; and whether or not patients feel that they have been properly listened to and understood. These and other non-specific components of the doctor-patient (or healer/shaman-patient) interaction can have surprisingly powerful effects. In a religious context, the apparent benefits of the equivalent of tablets and surgery (contact with religious authority figures; holy water, people or relics; pilgrimage and prayers, whether by the patient, the priest or others) are entirely due to placebo and non-specific effects but as in medical practice, the way in which religious interventions are perceived and delivered is a crucial variant. In both therapeutic and religious settings, style, presentation and, perhaps most important of all, symbolic meaning can make the difference between no benefit, or even a worsening of the symptoms, and dramatic improvements.

All treatment, like all religious practice, takes place in a particular context or setting. Medical, CAM and liturgical procedures involve belief systems that affect both patient and healer, parishioner and priest. To maximise placebo effects, the healer, medically qualified or not, must provide the right kind of placebo for that particular patient, just as, in a religious context, the priest must provide the right kind of religious ritual. Good placebo effects may be obtained by healers like me who knew that they were administering placebo injections or procedures but even better placebo effects may be obtained by healers who believe very strongly, but incorrectly, that they are administering a highly effective remedy. That is because they may communicate their completely unjustified enthusiasm to the patient. We all want our patients to get better and so do the patients themselves. This can easily lead to a mutual therapeutic delusion that is not always helpful.

Even when they don't realise that an intervention has no more than placebo effects, healers may administer it in a setting that maximises its non-specific effects and impressiveness to the patient. For example, wearing a white coat or a well-tailored suit in an expensively furnished clinic with lots of gleaming, bleeping, flashing, chrome-plated machines on display. Similarly, the placebo effects of religious procedures may be enhanced by the ecclesiastical equivalents of the distinguished consultant and the prestigious clinic: elaborate vestments, incense, emotive music in splendid churches and, as the visual analogue of chrome, lots of gold leaf on the reredos. Conversely, for some individuals and sects (Quakers, for example) the hallmark of a good church may not be 'bells, smells and vestments' but simplicity, plainness and frugality and the same principle applies to placebos. What soothes or impresses one patient may alarm another. (Why are all these machines and doctors here? Does that mean I'm very ill?)

What is it that makes so many people strongly believe in the non-existent specific healing powers of certain religious and CAM procedures, and of several conventional medical procedures that have no specific effect? All of us are placebo-responders, even Richard Dawkins, as we shall see, and therefore unlike some 'new atheists', I don't find the continued existence of religious people, placebo-responders and CAM supporters either surprising or a perpetual affront. That's just as well because all of them are going to be with us for a very long time and for much the same reasons. My approach to them in this book is essentially anthropological. Some of my friends are believers in religion and/or CAM. Many more religious believers have been my patients and I think I understand this large and important group of people reasonably well, especially when they are forced to contemplate the dark realities of disease and death. If I criticise some organised religions more than Margaret Mead and Bronislav Malinowski criticised the stone-age Melanesian societies that they studied as anthropologists, it is mainly because the shamans of the Trobriand Islands never claimed moral superiority over other tribes or at least didn't try to inflict their versions of morality and history on millions of other people, unlike their equivalents in Canterbury, Mecca and Rome. However, religion as a cultural, psychotherapeutic, social, tribal, charitable and mutual support institution is different from religion as truth-claim. In these roles, it is generally more benign and still has helpful and important functions for many people. Alain de Botton is one of several modern philosophers who argue that our secular society has not managed to come up with equally popular, accessible and, in ways that are sometimes therapeutically important, effective alternatives.[10] In the decade after the Soviet revolution, Communism tried and failed.[11]

Many people really "cannot bear very much reality" and as the philosopher Roger Scruton correctly noted, "the consolation of imaginary things is not imaginary consolation" but imaginary consolation can sometimes be dangerous as well as consoling. And dangerous, like opium and alcohol, precisely because it is consoling. In the developed world, most of the proletariat Karl Marx had in mind, when he referred to the opium of religion, no longer live in absolute poverty, squalor and the daily fear of illness and death but personal, economic or existential fears and anxieties remain common. Some prominent modern anxieties (about body-image for example) seem to be much more prevalent than they used to be. If reality is an uncomfortable place, many people will gladly move to a less demanding country of the mind. Until about 1920, when insulin became available, most medicines, like most folk remedies, really were no better than placebos. Many actually made the outcome worse than if the healers had given completely inert and inactive preparations. Medicine matched religion in its provision of comforting delusions and rituals. Modern medicine provides fewer delusions and more real good news. Religion does not. Here's another way of putting it: for most of recorded history, there was hardly any real progress or improvement in Western medical treatments and Eastern ones weren't much better. In the 17th century, quinine-containing fever-bark from South America began to be used in Europe for malaria, where it was helpful but also for every other fever, where it wasn't helpful because neither doctors nor folk healers understood that fever is caused by many different viruses, bacteria and parasites, the existence of which would not be known until several centuries later. In the 18th century, James Lind discovered, after one of the first controlled trials, that citrus juices could cure scurvy and Edward Jenner discovered vaccination, though a similar procedure had been used in the Ottoman Empire and other Eastern lands. Apart from those improvements, an 18th century European or North American physician was really no better than a 17th, 16th, 15th or even a 5th century one (AD or BC).

Apart from their ineffectiveness, another problem with ancient medicines was that the people who created them seemed to believe that increasing the number of ingredients in a given medicine would correspondingly increase its effectiveness. The classic example is Theriac, an elaborate preparation of opium that contained up to sixty separate ingredients. Some of them came from distant countries and were therefore expensive. The inclusion of gold also added to its cost, which naturally increased its placebo effects. With so many chemicals floating around, the risks of toxicity or of one chemical counteracting another were significant. If this book had been illustrated, one of the photographs would have shown a beautiful reliquary, currently in one of Rome's ancient churches, containing fragments of bone, skin or other relics of some two hundred saints - a religious version of Theriac.

A few other vaccines started to appear in the late 19th century but real pharmacological progress only became impressive in the 20th, when every decade brought real improvements and the pace of discovery continues to increase. If I were to move the vignettes of Gerald and Henri back a couple of thousand years, the only noticeable change would be in the different clothing and language of the characters. The medicines would probably have had different ingredients and the prayers and sacred objects would have been employed in the service of different gods but all would be equally devoid of specific therapeutic effects against the disease in question. With very few exceptions, surgery, apart from the management of accidents and wounds or small skin lesions, was little better before the mid-19th century anaesthetic and antiseptic revolutions. As for obstetrics, despite the invention of obstetric forceps in the early 1600s, you can get an idea of its limitations not just from the high maternal and child mortality rates of the time or a tour of old churchyards but from the melancholy fact that the royal obstetrician, Sir Richard Croft, shot himself in 1817 after Princess Charlotte and her baby died in childbirth.

Some personal history may help to explain my interest in placebos and to illustrate the importance of cultural and other non-specific factors. In the late 1960s, I spent a couple of enjoyable years working my way around the world as a doctor. In Melbourne, I was quickly approached by the GP of the friends with whom I was spending Christmas. He was desperate to take his family on holiday and hoped I could run his single-handed inner-city practice for a couple of weeks. Before leaving, he gave me a few useful tips about the patients and the area and when it came to one feature of the practice, he was very emphatic. Melbourne, at that time, had many first-generation immigrant families from Italy and Greece, who naturally brought with them not only their hopes and skills but also their tribal customs and beliefs. If I were called out by a Greek or Italian family to see a baby or indeed any child aged less than about seven, the families would expect me, he said, to give it an injection. This was very important and even if I didn't think that any medication was indicated, I should not fail to take out a syringe and plunge the needle into the child's flesh. If I failed to do this, they would simply call another doctor who would oblige them. Whether I chose to inject anything more potent than sterile water or saline was a decision that he was happy to leave entirely to me. Obviously, there would be cases where an antibiotic would be definitely or probably indicated but it was pointless, he said, to try to tell these families that antibiotics are not usually helpful for minor viral infections and can have undesirable side effects for both the child and the community. Or that oral antibiotics would usually be just as effective.

Needing no encouragement to accept the power of the placebo, I cheerfully did as he suggested. Many were the anxious mothers whose tears turned to smiles as I injected a cubic centimetre of the purest saline into their *bambini*. Many were the cups of dark coffee and glasses of grappa or ouzo that were pressed on me, during home visits, for these benevolent and beneficial deceptions. And relatively few, in consequence, were the *bambini* to whose minor and transient virus-induced miseries were added the far from minor discomforts of antibiotic-induced rashes or diarrhoea. A few years before this Melbourne experience, my first GP locum in Britain was in a practice so rural and so far from the nearest pharmacy that it dispensed most of the prescriptions on site, thus facilitating several simple therapeutic deceptions. In the days before gastric and duodenal ulcers were virtually abolished with what are now over-the-counter medicines, a standard treatment for ulcers and indigestion was a white mixture, usually labelled 'The Mixture', containing simple antacids and some flavouring. Before disappearing in the ambulance for what turned out to be his final heart attack, the GP, like his Melbourne counterpart, gave me some very specific placebo advice. If the white mixture seemed not to be working, I should simply add a little green dye, reassure the patient that this was a more potent version and relief would often follow. If relief didn't follow or didn't last long, I could repeat the process with a few crystals of potassium permanganate that turned it an impressively episcopal purple. Many GPs still do manage to prescribe placebos but as well as unnecessary vitamins, they give unnecessary and sometimes toxic antibiotics instead of the saline injections that so pleased my Melbourne families. (I was puzzled by the number of well-nourished Australians receiving weekly vitamin injections until I realized that in the Australian fee-per-item health system, unnecessary weekly vitamin injections produced four times the income of monthly prescriptions for unnecessary vitamin tablets.)

Other families, patients and cultures may have entirely different views about the right sort of treatment for their afflictions. Some may believe that only medicines made from rare and costly herbs or animals from remote regions will really do the trick. The religious equivalent of such beliefs is a mind-set in the parishioner or the priest (or both) which insists that prayer or confession are not enough and need to be beefed-up by visiting a local shrine or, better, a distant shrine involving much trouble and expense to get there, in order to touch a holy relic. Many people like to hedge their bets. When my travels took me to Jamaica's excellent university hospital, I found that acceptance of conventional Western medical practice was high but also that many of our patients would sacrifice a chicken with the local Obeah Man (i.e. shaman) just to be sure.

The rest of the book will have a lot to say about disease, unhappiness, fear, death and blighted hope, so let's end this chapter with a joke. Two men are in a train, sitting opposite each other. One man is tearing sheets of paper into small pieces and throwing them at intervals out of the window. (When I first heard this joke, trains had windows that could be lowered like those in a car.)

First man. 'Why are you doing that?'
Second man. 'Because it keeps the elephants away.'
FM. 'But there aren't any elephants within thousands of miles'.
SM. 'Yes. It's very effective.'

Placebos in medicine and their equivalents in religion are the elephant joke writ very large but instead of elephants, they are supposed to keep away disease and misfortune. They have a lot in common with 'kissing it better' and Samuel Pepys's 'hare's foote'.

Chapter 2
Theatres of Blood
Placebo effects in surgery and religious procedures

The obvious approach to a more detailed examination of placebo and non-specific effects in medical practice would begin by looking at tablets, capsules and injections but I'll start with surgery instead. If we are comparing the placebo effects of religious activity with those of what doctors do, surgical interventions are more appropriate because they have more in common with what goes on at churches and shrines, the subject of the next chapter. In both cases, the expected benefits are usually delivered by people wearing special garments that set them apart from ordinary citizens. Both patients and parishioners (or pilgrims) may also wear special clothing and there is a lot of ritual. Surgeons often call the pre-operative scrubbing-up and gowning-up 'sterile ritual'. Medical students quickly learn that there is definitely a right way and a wrong way to put on sterile gloves and that doing it the wrong way invalidates the whole procedure. These days, there may be music as well, though it's more for the benefit of the surgical priesthood than for the patient unless the operation is being done under local anaesthesia. The place where it occurs is called the 'operating theatre' because operations used to be performed in front of audiences. They still are but both church services and surgical operations are now televised and the audiences are much bigger.

As we saw in *A cure for serpents*, doing a placebo operation for a patient who is desperate for relief and has great faith in surgery (or in a particular surgeon) can have remarkably positive and lasting effects. Taking part in something that the patient believes or hopes is therapeutic or 'healing' is a major and necessary component of the placebo effect and the more subjectively impressive the procedure, the greater the placebo effect. This is true for healer/shaman-patient relationships and equally true for religious practitioners and their flocks. Since surgery is about as impressive as treatment can get, we would expect there to be a large non-specific component in any apparent effectiveness but surgery was a late-comer to the philosophy of the placebo-controlled trial. That's not surprising. Surgery was often done as an emergency for injuries and acute illnesses like appendicitis or perforated gastric ulcers. That made organising controlled trials more difficult, especially for life-threatening conditions. Unlike prescribing a medicine, surgery involves a group of people, making it more difficult to achieve the necessary degree of 'blindness'. There are other obvious reasons why doing surgical RCTs can be a challenge. If surgery is done to stop bleeding from wounds or injuries, there is usually no alternative, which is why there never have been and probably never will be RCTs of surgery vs no treatment in that situation, just as there are no RCTs of surgery with and without anaesthesia. (There are no RCTs of parachutes either.[12]) Surgeons, even more than physicians, tend to be programmed to *do something* and sometimes, common sense, or tradition, does actually tell us the right thing to do.

Eventually, surgeons did get round to doing controlled trials that involved asking themselves sceptical questions and invoking the null hypothesis. With a couple of possible exceptions, their religious equivalents never did, even though some religious ceremonies are not free of risk. Ironically, these risks, from fasting, long and exhausting pilgrimages, quasi-hypnotic states, prolonged and frenetic dancing or epidemics among pilgrims may be particularly risky for those who are already in poor physical or mental health. Multiple deaths from fatal stampedes at crowded pilgrimage sites occur regularly.[13] Even meditation and 'mindfulness' can be hazardous. After 12 hours of intense Zen meditation and fasting in SE Asia, a young and previously healthy patient of mine developed a severe anxiety state of almost delusional intensity that took several months to resolve. He was not unique.[14]

Connoisseurs of surgical placebo effects recall the 1950s studies that examined the effects of diverting the small mammary arteries of the chest into the heart muscle in the hope of improving blood flow in coronary disease to prevent heart attacks. Most patients felt better but they improved just as much after a sham operation involving only a Pirajno-style superficial incision and no arterial manipulation.[15] A more recent version of the same idea involved laser treatment of the heart muscle. Again, many patients reported improvement after this impressive procedure but no more than after the same procedure with the laser, unknown to the patient, switched off.[16] The improvements were mainly in ratings of pain, which is subjective, rather than cardiac function, which is more objective. The same failure to out-perform a comparable placebo procedure for stable angina in non-emergency situations was found with another drama-rich procedure involving catheterization of the coronary arteries.[17]

Recent studies have looked at placebo effects in backache, a condition that is notorious both for its tendency to come and go and for the frequent involvement of psycho-social factors in onset, severity and outcome. As a newly-qualified orthopaedic house-surgeon, I often treated patients with acute and incapacitating back pain. Many were fit young men who thought it unmanly to show distress but were in obvious agony. It's not easy to stand there and do nothing when despite generous analgesia, physiotherapy or visits to an osteopath, someone has been off work with severe pain for several weeks. Doing controlled surgical trials in this situation is also not easy but modern, minimally invasive surgical techniques have made it easier to do them, especially in less acute back pain. Some of the results have been very revealing. In an ageing population, many people have back pain apparently related to osteoporosis (softening of the bones) and the progressive collapse of vertebrae, causing the typical bent appearance of old age. Pumping bone-cement into the crumbling vertebrae in the hope of propping them up and preventing further crumbling, a procedure called 'vertebroplasty', is a relatively simple procedure and to backache-afflicted patients, it sounds like a good idea. In fee-per-item health services, it sounds like a good idea to hospitals, surgeons and their accountants as well and it has become quite popular. True to the spirit of science, sceptical enquiry and the null hypothesis, orthopaedic researchers tried to find out how much of the considerable improvement that often follows this procedure is due to placebo and non-specific effects. The answer is that they account for a very large proportion. Patients who only had a small incision under local anaesthetic did as well as those who had the cement as well. "There were significant reductions in overall pain in both study groups at each follow-up assessment [but there was] no beneficial effect of vertebroplasty as compared with a sham procedure in patients with painful osteoporotic vertebral fractures, at 1 week or at 1, 3, or 6 months after treatment".[18] There were similar results in trials of keyhole surgery for arthritis of the knee.[19]

For reasons already discussed, the relatively few placebo-controlled surgery trials that have been done rarely involved acute, life-threatening conditions but the conclusions of an analysis of those few trials are clear. "About a half of the reviewed trials showed superiority of the surgical procedure over placebo intervention, but *the magnitude of the effect directly related to the crucial surgical element was generally small.* [my italics] The majority of the trials showed an improvement in the surgical group as well as in the placebo group, which would suggest that some surgical procedures may have a placebo effect and that some of the benefits of surgery are related to factors other than the crucial surgical element."[20] Or to put it another way, placebo and non-specific effects accounted for a larger proportion of the improvement than the specific surgical procedure. In the other half of the trials, the full surgical procedure was *not* superior to the sham operation but unsurprisingly, there were fewer "adverse events" (i.e. complications) following the sham procedures. While the authors of the analysis note that some of these negative trials led to changes of surgical practice, notably in the abandonment of mammary artery surgery and greater patient selectivity in the knee procedures, the back surgeons, and many of their patients, were very reluctant to abandon vertebroplasty. I imagine that when bloodletting and leeches finally became unfashionable, some older doctors were equally reluctant to abandon them; '*because, you see, the patients feel so much better after it*'.

Sufferers from chronic back pain often take their problem to non-medical or CAM healers instead of (or as well as) consulting orthopaedic surgeons. Some of these healers have much in common with religious figures and one group of them took part in a carefully designed randomised and placebo-controlled clinical trial. 'Spiritual healing' is not quite the same thing as conventional prayer, since the nature of the curative 'spirit' is not so cut and dried as when prayers are uttered in the name of the monotheistic god but it has many similarities, and both procedures involve a belief in the existence of forces that are allegedly unmeasurable by science. Fortunately, the alleged specific healing effects of these alleged forces can be easily measured, using standard RCT methods. When Prof. Edzard Ernst was appointed to the world's first chair of CAM at Exeter University (more about him and it later) that was the subject of one of his earliest studies when he learned, to his surprise and mine, that 'Spiritual Healers' were the largest single body of CAM practitioners in Britain. He set out to compare Spiritual Healing with appropriate placebo procedures using actors or real practitioners, in the case of face-to-face healing and booths that were either empty or contained a concealed practitioner, in the case of 'distant' healing.

Prof. Ernst wisely involved the spiritual healers themselves in the design of the trial, so that if the results were disappointing, they could not easily complain that the trial was unfair. Patients attending a clinic for chronic pain resistant to conventional medical treatment (of whom there is definitely no shortage) were the subjects. Chronic back pain was common. Many improved considerably, some even discarding their walking sticks and wheelchairs as at religious shrines but it made absolutely no difference whether the patients were treated by 'genuine' healers or by actors. Booths containing healers obtained the same improvements as booths that contained only air.[21] It is against this sort of dramatic and symbol-infused background that all claims of healing – religious, CAM and conventional but especially religious and CAM - should be judged. Partly because of this study, I suggest, later in the book, that with relatively little training, some of the numerous 'resting' actors might be effectively employed as therapists in placebo research.

If pain and disability are strongly affected by the psychological and cultural factors that underlie placebo and non-specific effects, so is erectile function. Most adult male readers will know from personal experience that the presence of crying babies, the likelihood of being overheard or observed, cramped conditions or various aesthetic factors can seriously impair potency, just as the right ambience or a pleasant shared aesthetic experience can enhance it. Decreased potency and interest become common with increasing age. Some men don't mind this or even welcome it but many do. Viagra is significantly more effective than placebo but before Viagra, numerous drugs were claimed, mostly without good evidence, to strengthen both desire and erections and so were some surgical procedures. One of those was vasectomy and one of its most enthusiastic endorsements came from the aged Irish poet William Butler Yeats. That may now seem surprising. Millions of men have had a vasectomy since it became a common contraceptive method in the 1960s. Freedom from the fear of causing an unwelcome pregnancy removes an important cause of sexual performance anxiety and can therefore presumably improve potency in some cases but I think we would have heard by now if vasectomy commonly caused the dramatic increase in desire and potency that Yeats claimed it had done for him.[22] Eugen Steinach, an Austrian surgeon, initially promoted *unilateral* vasectomy, not for contraceptive reasons but in the mistaken belief that it would lead to greatly increased testosterone levels. Testosterone does increase slightly after bilateral vasectomy but only within the normal range, which is quite wide; typically between 250 and 1000ng/dL. It seems unlikely that Yeats's subsequent infatuation with Margot Ruddock had anything to do with the physiological effects of the operation and highly likely that it was due to placebo and non-specific effects; including one of those spontaneous changes for better or worse that occur in so many areas of human activity and interest without any obvious cause or explanation. Both sham surgery and sham injections usually have larger placebo effects than sham tablets but they all work in exactly the same way.

Chapter 3
The empty cassock
Placebo priests and placebo healers

For people who attend churches, the drama, ritual and theatricality of the services is an important part of the overall attraction. That's also true for many of the priests who perform at these events, especially High-Church Anglicans and the traditionalist wing of Roman Catholicism, but 'charismatic' sects often have rituals derived from an African or Afro-Caribbean background. Priests and parishioners can get very worked-up about even seemingly trivial details of liturgical practice in their churches, and at various times in the history of Christianity, Puritan and literally iconoclastic worshippers have removed, painted-over or destroyed images, statues and church ornamentation. Islamic Puritans are no different, the demolition of the giant Buddha statues at Bamiyan and the destruction of ancient tombs and manuscripts at Timbuktou being recent examples. Others complained or rebelled when those much-loved decorative or symbolic features were threatened or removed. It is in the nature of ritual that, at one level, it needs no explaining or justification. By their very familiarity, familiar rituals reassure people and make them feel comfortable. "Believe me", says one of Roald Dahl's characters, "there's nothing like routine and regularity for preserving one's peace of mind".[23] Conversely, deviations from the usual rituals can make people uncomfortable or angry and this happens even if the ritual in question has no particular function beyond its performance.

This tendency for ritual to ossify may increase when the ritual is part of a process that is supposed to bring benefits to those taking part in it. In a religious context, prayers may have to be recited in a particular way if they are to be perceived as efficacious, just as Pepys's hare's-foot needed a particular number of joints. Often, 'magic numbers' (typically multiples of three or seven) are involved. When a religious ritual is performed for overtly therapeutic purposes, as opposed to getting a better deal in the afterlife, correct performance is even more crucial.

The philosopher Roger Scruton, already quoted and no great friend to active atheism, notes that: "In all places and times, people have believed that there is a way into the eternal, a door out of time into a place where nothing changes and all is at rest within its being. And the key to this door is repetition. That is what sacred rituals, sacred words, and sacred places provide: the prayers, chants, costumes, steps and gestures that must be repeated exactly, and for which there is no explanation other than that this is how things are done".[24] You will have noticed that God is absent from Scruton's description. Alain de Botton, atheist though he is, feels that "Secular society has been unfairly impoverished" by the loss of these and other practices. "We are presented with an unpleasant choice between either committing to peculiar concepts about immaterial deities or letting go entirely of a host of consoling, subtle or just charming rituals for which we struggle to find equivalents in secular society".[25]

Of course, for many people, 'getting a better deal in the afterlife' is not a trivial matter and the correct performance of 'the prayers, chants, costumes, steps and gestures that must be repeated exactly' can be very important. The wording of a dedicatory plaque in the excellent private Catholic general hospital where I used to admit my alcoholic patients for discreet detoxification makes this very clear:

> In accordance with the wishes of the late Lord and Lady Brampton, the west wing of this hospital is always to be called and known as
> 'THE LORD AND LADY BRAMPTON WING'
> and the Catholic inmates of this wing and the nuns in charge thereof shall once every day recite aloud the 'Our Father' and 'Hail Mary' and also, at least on one day in each week for all time, say the 'Litany of the Holy Name' for the repose of the souls of Lord and Lady Brampton.[26]

Lord Brampton was a high court judge and a late convert to Catholicism. He was also, it seems, extremely worried about what might lie in store for him after he died and equally worried that the relevant protective rituals might not be performed in exactly the right way. This is very similar to the importance attached by homoeopathic practitioners to the ritual of 'succussion' (i.e. the hitting of containers of homoeopathic solutions against a leather cushion exactly one hundred times) in the preparation of their remedies, discussed later in the book. There is no rationale to the process or evidence for its relevance but the homoeopathic literature insists that proper succussion and therapeutic success are causally linked and the websites of leading homoepathic pharmacies lay as much stress on following the correct homoeopathic rituals as Lord Brampton did for the rituals of his own faith. The pharmacy texts of pre-1920s conventional medicine devoted the same sort of attention to the correct preparation of pharmaceuticals that, as we have seen, were nearly always ineffective and sometimes positively toxic. Lord Brampton might have felt confident that the nuns and the Catholic patients would recite the soul-preserving prayers and litanies in the right way but history suggests that in one important respect, his confidence might have been completely unjustified, since it is clear that those doing the praying sometimes have absolutely no faith in the deity to which they appear to pray. Like the actors in the RCT of spiritual healing, they may simply be walking placebos, though walking (and talking) placebos can be even more powerful than inanimate ones.

When clergy lose their faith, they do not necessarily leave or lose their clerical employment. A study by Daniel Dennett and Linda LaScola[27] asked the question: what is it like to be a pastor who stays the course in this situation? One short answer (not much discussed in their paper) is that from the point of view of their parishioners, it makes no difference – particularly if the priest keeps his doubts to himself. Leaving aside those primitive societies where the roles of priest and physician are combined in the witch-doctor or shaman, the roles of the modern priest and the modern physician often overlap. Both doctors and priests spend much of their lives demonstrating that a problem shared is often a problem halved, or at any rate a problem reduced. Both are walking placebos but whereas modern doctors are rather more than that, priests – ancient or modern - are not. Provided that he or she looks like a priest, talks like a priest and acts like a priest, neither parishioners nor other priests will be able to detect a priest who lacks what in theory ought to be a crucially important qualification for the job; the possession of a specific religious faith. Though I argue that no priest has more than placebo effects when praying, a disbelieving cleric can be regarded as a sham priest for comparative purposes.

The doubting American priests interviewed by Dennett and La Scola come across as a rather sad bunch, partly because they were doing a job that made them increasingly uncomfortable but mainly because most of them had nobody with whom they could share their sadness and discomfort. The interviews with researchers were often the first time they had been able to do that. There were only five of them in the study and they came from churches ranging from Southern Baptist through Methodist to Presbyterian but all insisted that they were not alone and were simply the tip of a very large and rarely-mentioned theological iceberg. (The recently-founded Clergy Project, 'a confidential online community for current and former religious professionals without supernatural beliefs' already had 636 members as of 2015, 172 current and 464 former priests. In the US, they come from nearly all states, including the Bible Belt.[28]) Most wanted to leave their posts but wondered what they would do instead and how they would make an equally comfortable living, especially if they lived in a church-owned house. Some couldn't even come out to their spouses and children. One Methodist pastor who went public, Tim Prowse, admitted that "As an active minister, I did not discuss my atheism with colleagues or parishioners. Facing lost wages, housing and benefits, I chose to remain silent. However, I did confide in my wife who provided a level of trust, understanding, and support that proved invaluable. Unfortunately, some ministers do not enjoy mature confidants".[29] Happily for him, friends offered him cheap housing and a job.

That was not an option for the first recorded Christian priest to say publicly and in print (or at any rate, in manuscript) that the whole thing was essentially a myth, that the Bible was man-made and full of contradictory and unpleasant stories and that religion had been co-opted by ruling elites to consolidate their hold over the plebs. That he is so little known probably reflects the fact that it has taken nearly 300 years for his only work to be recently translated into English. None of the 'new atheists' has mentioned him and he didn't appear in *Atheism: A Rough History of Disbelief*, Sir Jonathan Miller's short 2004 TV series. (When it was broadcast in the USA, the shocking word 'atheism' was removed from the title.) Jean Meslier's neglect by historians is surprising because as well as apparently being only the second European since Roman times to put his name to an overtly atheist document, Meslier was also unusual in being an early agrarian socialist and anti-monarchist like his near-contemporaries the Levellers of the English Civil War, though he doesn't mention them. (The first, as I only discovered shortly before this book went to press, was a Polish nobleman, Kazimierz Łyszczyński, but he was a philosopher, not a cleric.) Furthermore, Meslier's ecclesiastical credentials were impeccable, since he passed his entire adult life as the apparently popular priest of Étrépigny, that tiny village in North-East France mentioned in the Introduction, and knew exactly what he was rejecting. At some personal cost, he supported his downtrodden and impoverished parishioners against the local tyrant De Toully – a rapacious wicked squire straight out of central casting. Too scared to speak his mind to anyone during life, in 1729 he left by his death-bed three copies of a mordant, well-referenced denunciation of supernatural beliefs. He called it a *Mémoire* of his thoughts and sentiments about the religions of the world but it is often referred to as his *Testament.* "All religions are nothing but errors, illusion and imposture" is a typical chapter heading. "The wisdom and learning contained in the so-called holy books are only human" is another. To read Father Meslier is to read an earlier, hayseed incarnation of Richard Dawkins, Sam Harris and Christopher Hitchens. There's nothing new about the 'new atheists'.

Despite his small library and apparent lack of intellectual company, he criticised the numerous errors and inconsistencies in the Bible well before German theologians got round to it over a century later and over two centuries before Catholics were officially allowed to, in 1943. "What certainty do we have that the four Gospels ... were not corrupted and falsified, as we see happen to so many other books even today?" We also find proto-evolutionary thinking (Nature "acts blindly...without knowing what it is doing or why it is doing it") - even some proto-Malthusian anxieties. All very modern, as is his defence of divorce when domestic strife makes children miserable and parents "give them bad examples every day and fail to educate them...in the arts and sciences as well as in good manners". Meslier himself had a young 'housekeeper' (he passed her off as a cousin) and evidently had relaxed views about sex. Though not a vegetarian, he deplored the prevalent brutality towards farm animals.

His neglect may also be due to another dangerously heretical book titled 'Common Sense', wrongly attributed to Meslier since the 1790s and still confusingly published under his name. In some ways, 'Common Sense' is better written but its real author was an amiable aristocrat, the Baron d'Holbach, who wisely published everything pseudonymously and almost certainly rejected Meslier's radicalism, which was briefly recognised during the Revolution that followed d'Holbach's perfectly-timed death in 1789. In contrast, Voltaire said that Meslier wrote "like a carthorse". It's true that Meslier can be repetitious but there are several flashes, though his most famous (and invariably mis-attributed) phrase – "I would like to see the last king strangled with the guts of the last priest" - is not his own, as he truthfully records. In 1761, Voltaire published, I'm sorry to report, a dishonest and much-shortened travesty of the *Mémoire* that made Meslier appear a deist, like Voltaire himself. It excised all reference to Meslier's anti-monarchism and egalitarianism, both of them absolute anathema to Voltaire, presenting him as a death-bed convert rather than the life-long unbeliever he had undoubtedly been.

Meslier's parishioners knew nothing of his heretical views and neither did his priestly neighbours, nor his superiors. The local Archbishop, down the road at Reims, rapped his knuckles when he preached against the rapacity of Squire de Toully but records of parish inspections confirm that in all other respects, he was regarded even by Reims as a good and well-organised priest, in an age when the village priest was an important provider not just of spiritual comforts and rituals but also of official pronouncements and news. One thing that I find rather endearing about Meslier is that despite his rejection of religion, he seems to have enjoyed his pastoral work which, in the absence of a welfare state, must have been much more comprehensive than anything a modern village priest has to contemplate. I think of him as a bit like an old-fashioned country doctor – a Dr Finlay figure, knowing almost everything that went on in the village and possibly the only really literate inhabitant. His neat entries in the parish register indicate a sound education and confirm the authenticity of the *Mémoire* manuscripts in the Bibliothèque Nationale. We can easily imagine what went through his mind as he intoned every day the words of the mass and of all the other services – baptisms, weddings and funerals – that were so central to village life. Especially funerals, for the post-mediaeval 'Little Ice Age' reached one of its peaks during Meslier's tenure. The winter of 1708-9 was probably the coldest on record and over half a million died of famine in France alone. In Venice, people skated on the lagoon and as if what was known in England as 'The Great Frost' wasn't enough of a disaster, 1709 also included the War of the Spanish Succession. The site of Marlborough's famous victory at Oudenaarde is an hour's drive from Étrépigny today, just over the Belgian border. Even in happier periods, "a provincial economy within a hundred miles of Paris [in the mid-18th century] was a precarious balance between subsistence and dearth, with its agricultural technique hardly changed at all since mediaeval times".[30]

As it happens, we know exactly what Meslier thought about Holy Communion, the most solemn and impressive bit of theatre and audience-participation in the whole, impressive business of the Mass, because he tells us. *"Le dieu de pâte et farine",* he writes dismissively. "The god of dough and flour". Another 21st century Meslier – an unbelieving American priest who regularly blogs under the name of 'Stan Bennett' – describes his own feelings in church. "But while I like to study and think, the Sunday morning presentation fills me with dread because at some point, I'm going to be saying something I don't believe. My whole life, I have tried to be truthful, and now I am intentionally saying something I don't believe is true. This is what causes my heart to race, my blood pressure to rise, and bones to ache... I no longer speak of developing a personal relationship with Jesus, but instead speak of being loyal to his cause, which might include social justice issues as well as concepts of love, truth, and generosity."[31] Asked during the same interview if he ever got any interesting or challenging questions after his Easter sermons, he replied: "I never have seen much of that. They don't want me to rock their boat too much and force them to think because it might ruin their day. They expect me to use the religious language to which they are accustomed. Beyond the ritualism, it's not real to most of them. Actually, it's hard to disturb them because they aren't listening. ...And they'll crowd into one pew, sing the same songs as when they were young, watch the latest crop of children get baptized, smile at each other, and none of them will be able to repeat even a word or two of what I said, except maybe the funny story I told or an old thought that resonated from their Sunday school days."

A similar survey of rabbis who no longer believed in God found less unhappiness and more adaptation.[32] One, approaching retirement, even hoped that "he will be able to preach what he believes, and inspire others to adopt his beliefs. He is nearly certain that by then (7 years hence) he will have enough 'credit' with the members of his congregation that they will see religion - Judaism - the way he does, a human-social construct that provides comfort, support and companionship, regardless of and separate from a belief in a god". Another, reared and trained in Israel, lost his Ultra-Orthodox faith after being "slowly exposed to European atheism. He saw happy, loving people who were Godless. In his upbringing, this was not possible. The Godless were sinners, worse than those who did not practise." The author of the study, himself a rabbi working in Israel, concludes that in contrast to many forms of Christianity, "In as much as Judaism places a great emphasis on communal deeds rather than cultural creed, the rabbis still feel comfortable functioning in communities, school settings and informal educational roles." As yet, no Muslim academic seems to have been brave enough or optimistic enough to question Mullahs and Imams in a similar way. Physicians who don't believe in science - homoeopaths, for example - will do a lot of damage if you let them treat your hyperthyroidism homoeopathically, even if they look and sound to you like real doctors; but Roman Catholic priests who don't believe in God and think that communion wine is just wine can be absolutely indistinguishable in their rituals and the earthly results of their ministrations from the real thing. This is placebo effect with real style.

I don't know what the official Vatican line is on the validity of Holy Communion performed by apostates with bread and wine that they have supposedly consecrated, though apparently the actual words still do the trick even if the speaker has doubts. The Anglican church says that the sacraments "are not rendered ineffectual by the unworthiness of the minister" because "they do not do these things in their own name but in Christ's and minister by His commission and authority"[33] but what happens if 'unworthiness' means not sexual or financial misbehaviour but a fundamental rejection of Christ's existence, genealogy or authority? Were Meslier's deceived parishioners automatically excluded from heaven? It seems that having an unbelieving and privately blasphemous priest made no difference to their daily lives as compared with neighbouring parishes served by conventional and conforming priests. If there had been any obvious differences between Étrépigny and its neighbours as regards infant mortality, fertility, longevity, the incidence of common childhood and adult diseases and the health of its flocks and crops, I think the locals would have noticed and commented. The same presumably goes for Stan Bennett's parishioners, except that today's detailed mortality and morbidity statistics would have revealed any differences even more quickly. Epidemiologists would soon descend on any town or suburb with unexpectedly large or small numbers of patients with particular diagnoses, or of deaths.

We certainly know, as Meslier did, what that official Vatican line was when it came to unbelievers themselves, because he mentions a particularly horrifying example that occurred only a few decades before his birth. Lucilio Vanini, who sometimes called himself Julio Cesare Vanini, was a well-connected itinerant academic from a prosperous Italian family – a sort of Alain de Botton of his time. He had a lively and irreverent writing and lecturing style but his contacts with the movers and shakers of Parisian society kept him out of trouble until 1619. In that year, a book that he had written came to the attention of some of the ecclesiastics and magistrates of Toulouse when he was staying in the area. It was written in the form of a Socratic dialogue and did not advocate atheism but one of its fictional characters discussed the forbidden topic in an oblique and almost apologetic way. That was too much for the defenders of the status quo who convicted him of atheism and blasphemy. Vanini managed to give a brave little speech before his tongue was cut out and he was strangled and burned to ashes aged only 33. In Warsaw in 1689, similar barbarities were inflicted on Łyszczyński, although after his tongue was torn out, he was beheaded before being burned. His atheist treatise, *De non-existentia Dei* (On the non-existence of God) was burned with him. Even when they had less barbaric deaths, that sort of heretic was often buried in an unmarked grave, as Meslier was when his *Testament* was quickly discovered and read – the Vatican equivalent of Moscow's air-brushing of dissident communists from the official record.

Chapter 4
Mesmerising moments
Charisma and consciousness in churches and consulting-rooms

When healers and priests are thought to be particularly good at their job, they often attract the adjective 'charismatic'. Apart from its specifically religious meaning ('a divinely bestowed power or talent') dictionary definitions of charisma include "Compelling attractiveness or charm that can inspire devotion in others" and "charm, presence, aura, personality, force of personality, strength of character, individuality; magnetism, animal magnetism, drawing power, attractiveness, appeal, allure, pull; magic, spell, mystique, glamour".

In practice, what it means is that charismatic people have an unusual ability to lift the mood and inspire hope in a happy ending together with belief that they have some special gift. In times of war, men under the command of charismatic officers and NCOs typically claim that they would have followed them anywhere, though it is in the nature of warfare that it is mainly the victorious or the lucky who survive to make such claims. Unfortunately for both professions, some of the greatest frauds and villains as well as some of the most respected healers and priests have been very charismatic individuals. Several even managed to earn a place in both categories. Usually, charisma is a personal characteristic but sometimes, it seems to go with the office. Royal visits cheer and energise all but the most moribund or anti-monarchist hospital patients, even if the visitors hardly speak a word to them. Priests and doctors still rank among the most respected professions and it is a fortunate fact of medical life that patients will often do things for their doctors that they would not do for their spouses or employers, or for themselves. I am sure this is true of priests as well and even when doctors don't wear distinctive clothing (as most GPs and psychiatrists don't) we often wear invisible priestly robes.

Considering how important charisma can be in the outcome of religious and therapeutic encounters, it is interesting that it seems never to have been systematically studied, even though like all human characteristics that can be observed or felt, it can be measured to some extent by using a simple 10-point Visual Analogue Scale (VAS), sometimes called a Lickert Scale. (1 = no charisma; 10 = lots of it.) Perhaps one reason is that any such study would be difficult to do without revealing embarrassing information about the different levels of charisma possessed by the clinicians working in the relevant institution. There is also the problem that one patient's charismatic healer may be another patient's smooth-talking con-man. Still, several famous historical healers were described by their biographers as charismatic, especially but by no means exclusively if they specialised in patients suffering from conditions that were essentially psychological, or from physical conditions that had a large psychological element. By those last three words, I don't mean conditions that were 'imaginary' or that were primarily 'caused' by psychological processes. What I do mean is that all patients with essentially physical conditions have underlying psychological or personality characteristics that for better or worse can strongly affect their perception of the condition and the amount of pain and distress it causes them. Among my case-histories are two patients with paralysed limbs who, for very different psychological reasons – none of them 'pathological' - were unusually cheerful. They had symptoms that would seriously worry most of us but it did not worry these patients so much because the symptoms had a different meaning for them. It should not be surprising if people with differing but still essentially 'normal' personalities are made unusually anxious, fearful or even suicidal by symptoms and disabilities that most people would cope with more easily. A classic and widely-understood example is the ambitious athlete who has a comparatively minor injury that does not interfere with normal life but is damaging or even fatal to his or her competitive ambitions. There are many other examples involving matters that were of crucial but unique importance to a particular patient and could only be understood if one knew important bits of their life history. However illogical, weird or even ludicrous some of these matters may seem, if they are important to the patient, they may turn out to be important for the doctor. When a patient is not responding to treatment in the expected way, the 'matters' may turn out to be an important part of the explanation. Sometimes, they are almost the whole explanation. Furthermore, as the earlier teddy-bear analogy illustrates, other unique and idiosyncratic factors can make placebo effects larger or smaller.

Until a generation or two ago, most GPs were well-placed to recognise or ferret out these factors because they often knew their patients well. They often knew the whole family too and sometimes even the employer. That sort of GP used to be common when I qualified but is now rather rare. Greater mobility of both patients and doctors makes continuity of care difficult except perhaps in country practices. Greater pressure on the time of GPs because of increased expectations and an ageing population makes it difficult to offer the unhurried consultations that may be the only way in which these factors can emerge. Even then, patients may need time to trust a doctor with sensitive, shameful, embarrassing or unlikely information. Private GPs, like private CAM practitioners, provide more time but they do not always know the family background. Charisma can shorten the process in two ways. First, the right sort of charisma may make it easier for patients to reveal things to doctors or even to admit things to themselves. Secondly, it can help patients to re-define their problems and their self-image in ways that are useful to them. I would be very surprised if similar considerations did not affect the priest-parishioner relationship as well.

Charisma may not have been systematically studied but we have a good description of the *modus operandi* of one charismatic back-pain specialist, Dr John Sarno, written by a psychiatrist attached to the same medical school campus. He was intrigued by his colleague's reputation for curing persistent back problems that had resisted the hospital's rheumatologists and orthopaedic surgeons and while he did not sit in on a real consultation, he invited Dr Sarno to give a teaching seminar and had several discussions with him. In a chapter entitled 'A shaman in the halls of medicine',[34] Prof Marc Galanter describes him as "a reserved, neatly dressed, slight man, not more than five and a half feet tall and apparently well into his 70s. He spoke in measured tones, hardly coming across as a firebrand...". Dr Sarno had a theory about the causes of back pain that guided his treatment – essentially tension due to "unconscious anger" arising from "[feelings of] inferiority due to mental abuse they have experienced at their parents' hands...the need to achieve perfection and thereby to be perceived as 'good' [and] life circumstances that build up resentment in people's minds". As Galanter comments: "His theory seemed somewhat speculative, although not unreasonable, but I could see that the way he presented it would not win him a following in the world of laboratory-based medicine". I too have doubts. According to a 2014 review, lower back pain "causes more disability globally than any other condition"[35] but it is not evenly distributed and is not over-represented in Japan, where perfectionism seems built in to the culture and where suicide among students who fail exams, like suicide in general, is high by global standards.

As to his clinical techniques: "He would speak with a potential patient on the phone for five minutes or so to see whether they might be amenable to his approach *and would turn down most people who called.* [my italics] If he accepted a patient, though, he would have them come in to spend an hour with him for a physical exam and a discussion of how he understood the nature of their back pain, essentially telling them what he had just told me. He said that this would be followed by the patient's attending his lectures". Some patients were also referred for more formal and general psychotherapy. (Dr Sarno favoured the Adlerian model.)[36]

Prof Galanter wondered "how Sarno's words could enter the minds of his patients and put their pain to an end. It just seemed that the calm conviction that he conveyed came through to his patients and somehow relieved them of the tension that they were feeling, tension that he said was causing the pain for which they had sought him out. There did seem to be some parallel to the way faith healers could relieve conversion symptoms such as hysterical blindness and falling mute, aided by the anticipation in their subjects of a miraculous cure". I share Prof Galanter's hope that "conventional medicine might be able to take advantage of the techniques of shamanic healers". The challenge is to use those techniques honestly and without deceiving ourselves about the real mechanisms involved.

I suggest that hypnosis can reasonably be viewed as an aspect of charisma. It wasn't part of the curriculum at my medical school but the student medical society could invite anyone it wanted to give a lecture and one of our invited speakers was a medical hypnotist – a conventionally trained doctor who also used hypnosis in some conditions. That's when I first realised that hypnosis is a rather impressive phenomenon with some interesting clinical and philosophical implications. During his presentation, he showed a short film of a patient who was having his appendix removed under hypnosis. This unusual anaesthetic technique was employed because the patient had previously been successfully hypnotised for some other reason and was evidently a 'good subject'. It was clear that no other anaesthetic was used because throughout the procedure, the patient was smoking a cigarette and showed no sign of pain or distress. I suppose the hypnosis could have been a fake and the operation actually done under local or spinal anaesthesia but the only person in the film who seemed at all uncomfortable was the operating theatre sister, who was literally wringing her hands with anxiety. She would hardly have done that if either of those anaesthetic techniques had been used since they are recognised alternatives. In any case, it wouldn't have made sense for the lecturer to mislead us if he was trying to increase our awareness of hypnosis. He stressed that not everyone could be hypnotised to this degree but suggested that hypnosis might have been more widely used for surgery had not ether and chloroform anaesthesia been discovered at about the time that James Braid was introducing hypnotic anaesthesia to Britain in the 1840s and James Esdaile was being taught how to use it by indigenous practitioners in Britain's Indian colonies.

I know several dentists who use hypnosis instead of (or in addition to) local anaesthetics for fillings and extractions. They say it is especially useful in children, who particularly dislike having needles stuck into their gums. Only once did I see hypnosis used in psychiatry, when an elderly locum consultant used his swinging pocket watch, Hollywood-style, to hypnotise an anxious out-patient who seemed to go to sleep for a while. When the consultant left the room briefly, I asked the patient what the experience had been like. "Well", he said, "I wasn't really asleep but he's a nice old boy and I didn't want to disappoint him". Despite this fiasco, I thought that hypnosis was a technique I ought to learn. I went on a couple of courses but never got the hang of it, possibly because it may require levels of thespian skill and simulated sincerity (much the same things, arguably) that don't come very easily to me.

The only patient on whom I tried to use hypnosis clinically was a gynaecologist from a Muslim country where female genital mutilation was routine in all classes. He had been married to a European woman and had no sexual difficulties then or during the occasional one-night stand but despite his Westernisation and sophistication, he was inhibited by his residual cultural loyalties from disobeying his mother back home when she informed him that since it was not right for him to be wife-less, she had found him a suitable local girl. As a gynaecologist, he was particularly familiar with the scarring that even mild female genital mutilation causes and he knew that after the traditional wedding ceremonies, it would be necessary to prove his potency by breaking through his new wife's scar tissue if necessary and leaving some blood on the bedsheets as a sign of success for the anxious mothers who would scrutinize them the next morning. The contemplation of this misogynistic barbarism (or 'cherished manifestation of cultural diversity' if you are a certain sort of post-modern sociologist) so unmanned and disconcerted him that he feared he would be unable to perform adequately on the wedding night but since he was due to fly home only a few days later, my treatment options were rather limited. I tried hypnotic suggestion but also gave him a prescription for Potensan Forte, the deluxe version of a popular and perhaps modestly effective pre-Viagra drug for erectile dysfunction. As well as having an extra ingredient or two, it was distinguished from the simpler and cheaper tablet – plain

Potensan – by being gold-plated, the last drug in the British pharmacopoeia to incorporate this fine old technique for enhancing placebo effects. I don't know if my efforts were successful but no postcard arrived from his homeland bearing a short but triumphant message. It seemed that I was not cut out to be a hypnotist but the phenomenon of hypnosis is real enough and it is obviously a purely psychological process.

To learn more about hypnosis and to see it in action, I contacted the stage and TV hypnotist Derren Brown. He invited me to watch one of his shows and to join him backstage after his performance. Among the many impressive examples of how ordinary people can be enabled to do extraordinary things, the one that impressed me the most involved a slim young woman and a large suitcase full of bricks that had been wheeled onstage on a trolley by two hefty assistants. Unhypnotised, she could not lift it. After brief hypnotic suggestion, she could. It seemed very similar to the amazing feats of strength that were often seen in cases of demonic possession. Some of Derren's other acts were more obviously therapeutic, as when people with assorted aches and pains reported that the pains had gone or were much reduced. To sceptics who might wonder, as I did before the show started, whether fraud or audience 'plants' would be involved, I can report that many of Derren's acts were preceded by such persuasive randomisation techniques as throwing a frisbee into the audience and asking the person who caught it to throw it again, the next recipient being then invited onstage. The bricks in the suitcase seemed genuine enough to the woman who was about to try to lift it and Derren assured me that they were. However, my main reason for believing that Derren was not deceiving us is that in several books and television discussions, he consistently tries to demystify his craft and to explain it, mostly using understandable terms and concepts from psychology and neurophysiology. He is also a paid-up, free-thinking sceptic and abandoned his fervent adolescent belief in the God of Evangelical Christianity to become a definite unbeliever in his twenties. Charisma radiates from him, possibly aided by his fast-talking style and instant repartee and a niceness and lack of evasiveness that seem as genuine as they are striking. As with placebos, his acts involve a measure of deception but he is honest about this kind of dishonesty, which is limited and task-related rather than general and intellectual. For the record, Derren thinks that one of his most remarkable achievements was enabling one of his subjects to immerse himself completely and cheerfully in ice-cold water for several minutes. You can watch it on YouTube.[37]

Derren says there are two schools of thought about the nature of hypnosis. One holds that it is a special state, distinct from the normal range of human perception. The other, which is his own view, regards hypnosis as part of that normal range and something that can be experienced by many 'ordinary' people given the right circumstances, as seems apparent from the behaviour of the randomly selected audience members who went onstage for some acts. (Others were self-selected.) It is also the view of Michael Heap of Sheffield University, an academic psychologist who has a special interest in hypnosis and its mechanisms.[38] "Hypnosis may be best conceived as a set of skills to be deployed by the individual rather than as a state". On the other hand, "...undertaking hypnosis as though the individual were indeed being placed into a special trance state may in some cases promote an effective outcome".

Whatever happens during hypnosis – and as a fairly recent brain scan study conceded: "The neural mechanisms underlying hypnosis and especially the modulation of pain perception by hypnosis remain obscure."[39] – it definitely involves suggestion by self and/or others, among several possible factors and definitely doesn't involve external chemicals or medications. Yet under hypnosis, things that would normally be very painful can happen without any apparent pain or any attempt to move the relevant part of the body away from the cause of the pain. In a therapeutic context, it doesn't matter if hypnosis simply makes people *believe* that they are not feeling pain when, at some level within the brain, they actually *are* feeling it. Studies of brain activity suggest that this may actually be what happens in hypnosis. The point is that if a combination of suggestion, culture and belief can *remove or diminish* pain and sensation, it can surely also *produce or increase* them and that goes a long way towards explaining – or at least validating – both psychosomatic symptoms and the undesirable and unpleasant *nocebo* effects that are the flip side of placebo effects and get a fuller discussion later. Suggestion and belief are at the heart of the placebo effect, at least in humans, and they can clearly have extremely powerful effects on other aspects of human thought and behaviour, including religious ones. I don't mean that the placebo effect is exactly the same thing as hypnosis; only that there are some very close and interesting similarities. Since hypnosis can cause impressive and therapeutically useful changes in feelings, emotion and behaviour, we should not be surprised if equally impressive and useful things happen because of placebo effects.

If people can have abdominal surgery under hypnosis without feeling pain, it is hardly surprising that hypnosis can achieve less dramatic forms of pain relief. An RCT of hypnosis vs simple relaxation for oral-facial pain[40] showed large differences for the hypnosis group compared with the relaxation controls. Relaxation involved different procedures compared with hypnosis but was very similar in terms of the amount and type of attention. Within the hypnosis group, "highly hypnotic susceptible patients had greater decreases in VAS pain scores...when compared to less susceptible patients". Another study involved bone marrow sampling, a rather unpleasant diagnostic procedure. Because it is needed for the diagnosis of leukaemia and for assessing treatment progress, and because acute leukaemia is mainly a disease of early life, bone marrow samples often have to be aspirated in childhood, usually from the breastbone. I have never been on the receiving end of the procedure but I have done it a few times and even with generous local anaesthetic preparation around the puncture site, the crunching sound as the wide-bore needle goes through the outer surface of the bone is not exactly relaxing for either party. Fortunately, a precise, well-defined and repeatable procedure such as this is relatively easy to study. In a randomised trial of hypnosis vs Cognitive-Behavioural coping skills and a 'no treatment' control group,[41] both treatments gave better results than no treatment and were equally effective in most respects but "children reported more anxiety and exhibited more behavioural distress in the CB group than in the hypnosis group". An even more impressive blinded RCT was done by the presumably hard-headed, no-nonsense cancer specialists at a major New York hospital. Women about to have their breast lumps biopsied were given either "a 15-minute pre-surgery hypnosis session conducted by a psychologist or nondirective empathic listening" – the latter to control for the amount of attention and personal contact that patients received. Despite needing significantly less general and local anaesthetic. the hypnosis group not only experienced considerably reduced levels of pain, nausea, fatigue and other unpleasantness but cost the hospital nearly 10% less than the $8500 average for the procedure "mainly due to reduced surgical time".[42] Even in the setting of a busy Casualty department, hypnosis requiring "only modest training" relieved acute pain that had failed to respond to large doses of a powerful opiate.[43] More impressive still is a report from a Belgian surgical unit of 121 operations on the thyroid and parathyroid glands without local or general anaesthesia and using only hypnosis with light 'conscious' sedation (meaning that patients were still able to respond to instructions). In no case was it necessary to revert to general anaesthesia and patient satisfaction was high. Interestingly, the surgeons reported less bleeding in what is often a delicate procedure in an area well-supplied with blood vessels, compared with a similar group where general anaesthesia was used.[44] Both placebo effects and hypnosis can have very powerful effects on feeling and function and they work through entirely psychological and neurophysiological processes intrinsic to humanity. The nature of those processes, still far from clear, is less important than their power.

My final example would be almost unbelievable had it not been published, with photographs, in the *British Medical Journal* by a trainee anaesthetist, Dr Albert Mason, working at the world-famous Queen Victoria Hospital in East Grinstead, south of London, where the plastic surgeon Sir Archibald McIndoe pioneered the treatment of badly-burned RAF pilots in WW2.[45] The patient was a boy of 16 who had been born with abnormal skin. It soon developed into a variant of the condition called icthyosis, which causes most of the body to be covered in rough, hard skin resembling thick fish-scales. By the time of his treatment, it had become "a black horny layer covering his entire body except his chest, neck and face ... To the touch, the skin felt as hard as a normal finger-nail, and was so inelastic that any attempt at bending resulted in a crack in the surface, which would then ooze blood-stained serum. In the skin flexures, there were fissures that were constantly being reopened by movement and were chronically infected and painful ... His schooling was interrupted because pupils and teachers objected to his smell". On two occasions when an area of skin was surgically excised, it grew back equally hard and scaly.

The young anaesthetist was interested in hypnosis and suggested a trial, to which his seniors agreed. To make it as sure as possible that any subsequent improvement was not just a spontaneous fluctuation in the disease process (though that would be very atypical) he hypnotized – if that is the right word – just one arm first. "Five days later, the horny layer softened...and fell off...The skin underneath became pink and soft...At the end of 10 days, the arm was completely clear from shoulder to wrist." Subsequently, the other arm and then the legs, separately, also responded to hypnotic suggestion, though the clearance was not quite as complete as with the arms. Several months later, the improvement had been maintained. His social handicaps removed, he became "a happy, normal boy, though still educationally retarded, and is already being employed as an electrician's assistant". It is surely inconceivable that a junior doctor would have submitted the report to such a prestigious and widely-read journal unless his senior colleagues had also seen the results. Indeed, he thanks the consultant who had clinical responsibility for the patient for permission to publish the report – as tradition demands. Even the pathologist who microscopically examined the excised tissue is named in the article. Furthermore, even if the improvement had not been so lasting, the dramatic, repeated changes in consecutive limbs and other areas defy any normal understanding of healing processes and suggest that the modest amount of serious research into hypnosis might usefully be increased. Ironically, young Dr. Mason subsequently became disillusioned with hypnosis and embraced psychoanalysis instead.

Just as some patients are more susceptible than others, so some hypnotists are better than others at obtaining the desired effects. Differing levels of hypnotic skill probably reflect differing levels of charisma, among other qualities but I cannot find any studies. However, unlike acupuncture or homoeopathy, hypnosis seems to be an intervention that requires specific rather than non-specific skills. Like surgical ability, hypnotic ability is not evenly distributed in society but like surgical skills, it is also both real and measurable, even if not often measured. I think hypnosis should therefore not be regarded as a typical CAM treatment, even if many of its practitioners currently work in that setting.

Mesmerism was an 18th century version of hypnotism and the verbs 'mesmerise' and 'hypnotise' are still synonyms for 'powerfully influencing someone' or 'to have someone's attention completely so that they cannot think of anything else'. In 1784, not long after James Lind's pioneering trial of treatments for scurvy, King Louis XVI of France set up a commission to submit the new craze for Mesmerism to the same process of scientific scepticism. The members, who included Benjamin Franklin and the distinguished chemist Lavoisier,[46] did a controlled study of individuals who were allegedly 'sensitive' to the supposed 'vital fluid' or 'animal magnetism' that Mesmer claimed to be able to incorporate into people and objects, another manifestation of the 'vitalism' that was fashionable at the time and that also influenced Samuel Hahnemann, the founder of homoeopathy. Like priests in religious ceremonies, Mesmer also exploited drama. He was "a theatrical virtuoso, employing costume (lilac robes) sound effects (the tones of a glass harmonica, whose ethereality spoke for that of the universe) and impressive props such as magnetic tubs."[47] Like priests, he also "recognized the social value of treatment in groups", though tastes differ and some patients do not like sharing their illnesses, hang-ups or guilty secrets with others. As well as confirming that the scepticism that was such an important feature of the Enlightenment now extended to medicine, the study showed that under the blind conditions that are characteristic of a sceptical, scientific approach to truth-claims, the alleged 'sensitivity' did not exist. These individuals fainted or had 'convulsions' (though not true epileptic convulsions) when in contact with material that they believed to have been 'magnetised', even when it hadn't been.[48] It was all a matter of suggestion, though how people react to suggestion depends to a large extent on how they have been programmed or conditioned to respond, whether by life experience (including religious indoctrination and belief), media reporting or by healers, especially if they have faith in them. A later 18th century study by Dr John Haygarth showed that 'Perkins Tractors', a briefly fashionable treatment similar to Mesmerism and using tongs made of metals supposedly crucial to their effectiveness, worked equally well when made of wood painted to look like metal. He published his findings under a title that says everything; *On the imagination as a cause and as a cure of disorders of the body, exemplified by fictitious tractors and epidemical convulsions.*[49]

There was much self-congratulation in religious circles about a study showing that compared with unbelievers, Catholics experienced less experimental pain when simultaneously shown an image of the Virgin Mary.[50] The then Bishop of Durham, the Rt. Rev. Tom Wright said: "The practice of faith should, and in many cases does, alter the person you are. It can affect the patterns of your brain and your emotions. So it comes as no surprise to me that this experiment has reached such conclusions." He was right, of course, but what he predictably failed to add (or perhaps to understand, which would be more worrying) was that the *nature and object* of that faith are irrelevant and non-specific. The results certainly didn't prove that faith in Christianity was the crucial variable and that comparable levels of faith in other religions or gods (or Hitler) wouldn't have had any beneficial effect. Photographs of ecstatic German faces when Hitler was driven through a town or addressed a gathering are not very different from the ecstatic faces of the faithful when a pope does the same thing.

A similar study showed that for patients with irritable bowel syndrome (IBS), a sham medical procedure - in this case a balloon inserted into the rectum but not inflated – also reduced pain significantly.[51] That could hardly have been more different from seeing an image of the Virgin Mary but *it had exactly the same sort of effects* and involved similar areas of brain activity. The Catholics had presumably been conditioned by their experiences and beliefs to be impressed by specific religious images. The IBS patients had presumably been conditioned by theirs to be impressed by what looked like (and presumably felt like) some sort of medical intervention. It shows yet again that the nature and meaning of a placebo are crucially important and that for maximum effect, they need to reflect the patient's or the parishioner's cultural, emotional, symbolic and intellectual experiences, tastes and expectations. They are important because it is clear that placebo and non-specific effects can be increased and individualised in ways that are simply not possible with specific pharmacological or surgical interventions, as already discussed.

An interesting slant on the pain-relieving properties of images of the Virgin appears in a review of cultural meanings and differences in placebo responses. It seems that Italy is an exception to the general finding that red placebos stimulate while blue ones have a calming effect but the exception applies only to Italian men. The author speculates that "Many Italian women have a special relationship with the Virgin Mary [who]...in religious art is almost always shown in blue". However, blue – *'azzuro'* – gives both a name and a colour to the national football team. Consequently, "Blue, for many Italian men, is not a colour of solace but of excitement and stimulation, of joy and madness...It is hardly the colour of sleep!"[52]

Where pain is concerned, simple cultural and environmental factors as well as placebo effects and hypnosis (including self-hypnosis, learned or instinctive) may explain why certain people at certain times have been able to tolerate apparently agonising procedures without showing signs of suffering severe pain. In some cultures, ritual male circumcision is delayed until adolescence and is part of a rite of passage to manhood. Being 'manly' in this context includes putting up with pain, so these adolescents generally manage to stay silent during the procedure. I once saw a TV interview with children aged about ten who had had their hands cut off in a West African civil war. They had been told that if they cried during the amputations, they would be killed, so they didn't cry. (Perhaps it was a 'survival effect' and they were a selected sample because those who did cry didn't live to appear on TV.) Louis XIV is said to have endured an operation for an anal fistula (no anaesthesia, obviously) without making a sound. Saint Ignatius Loyola, the founder of the Jesuits, suffered a fractured femur from a cannon-ball during a siege in his earlier life as a soldier. It healed eventually but was badly deformed and he apparently endured having it broken again and re-set without complaint, as he also did a little later when a projecting piece of bone was sawn off. My medical school was proud of being London's oldest hospital[53] (founded in 1102) and one of the sterile drapes used during operations was still called a 'stone cloth'. This referred to its original and decidedly unsterile use during the procedure of cutting into the bladder from below, from a point just in front of the anus, to remove bladder stones. Even though in good hands it might take little more than a minute or two, it must have been both terrifying and extremely painful but Samuel Pepys was 'cut for the stone' in March 1658. As far as we can tell from his Diaries, he was not psychologically scarred for life and it evidently did no harm to his well-documented libido. The stone was reportedly the size of a tennis ball – as in Real Tennis, not the modern, larger Wimbledon variety. Another pre-anaesthesia sufferer is said to have passed a nail down his urethra into his bladder and then used a hammer to hit the nail against the stone to break it into pieces small enough to be passed in his urine![54]

The Hunterian Museum of the Royal College of Surgeons in London has a description of the removal by John Hunter in 1785 of a benign tumour of the parotid gland (the salivary gland behind and under the lower jaw) that weighed 4kg. The operation took 25 minutes and the patient, John Burnley, "did not cry out during the whole procedure". Since breast cancer was both common and visible and thus a candidate for surgery, women also often submitted to the knife. The 18th century diarist Fanny Burney described in words that are not for the squeamish how she felt the scalpel scraping against her ribs during the excision of a tumour.[55] Perhaps our forebears were more accustomed than we are to the idea that severe pain is something that we may simply have to grin and bear - or just bear - when it happens.

Moving several thousand miles to the east, we find descriptions of Indian widows who, in the ritual of *suttee* (or *sati*), threw themselves onto the funeral pyres when their recently dead Hindu husbands were cremated. Many European commentators mentioned the remarkable absence of screams, or even anticipatory anxiety. A 17th century French traveller reported that a Muslim ruler, trying to dissuade "an attractive 22-year old woman" who sought his permission to commit *suttee*, pointed out the particular agonies of death by burning. She called, contemptuously for a lighted torch to be brought and held her hand in the flame, then "pushed in her arm up to the elbow, till it was immediately scorched", all "without the least grimace". In 1823, a Times correspondent in India reported that the pulse of a widow he had unsuccessfully tried to dissuade from *suttee* was "far calmer than my own at the moment of writing".[56]

I suspect that these remarkable but credible stories of culturally-induced or self-induced insensitivity involve mechanisms similar to those of hypnosis. Cultural and other quasi-religious beliefs can even affect the date of death, if not its inevitability. A study intriguingly titled 'The Hound of the Baskervilles effect'[57] aimed to find out "whether cardiac mortality is abnormally high on days considered unlucky: Chinese and Japanese people consider the number 4 unlucky, white Americans do not". After examining "All Chinese and Japanese (n=209,908) and white (n=47,328,762) Americans whose computerised death certificates were recorded between the beginning of January 1973 and the end of December 1998", they found very significant peaks for cardiac deaths on the fourth day of each month for Oriental-Americans but no similar peak for the others.

Chapter 5
Shocked to the Core
The power of placebo electro-convulsive therapy

Electro-Convulsive Therapy (ECT or, in the USA, Electro-Shock Therapy) has had a bad press. For many people, reading or seeing 'One flew over the cuckoo's nest' evoked an image of a psychiatric patient being held down on a trolley, having electrodes applied to his head and then going into spasms. It does involve passing electricity through the brain and can easily be made to look like torture, though for many years it has always been given under a general anaesthetic. For those who are interested and not too squeamish, there is a short history of the introduction of ECT at the end of this chapter. In the 1960s and 70s when Dr R D Laing, Dr Thomas Szasz and the anti-psychiatry movement were at their zenith, and when 'Cuckoo' was made into a film, ECT was routinely denounced as barbaric. The ideologues who denounced it weren't noted for their knowledge or concern about the comparative effectiveness of various treatments but if you had asked them, they would probably have told you that ECT was not only barbaric but also ineffective. It didn't help its defenders that around that time, one of the several scandals involving some of the old British asylums revealed that ECT patients were occasionally dragged protesting to the place of electrocution and the analogy of the electric chair was a bit too close for comfort. To the man or woman in the street, it must have seemed obvious that plugging people into the mains is harmful. Most of us have experienced electric shocks and everyone knows that electricity can be lethal. Surely ECT fries your brain?

There are psychiatrists who never use ECT and patients who would never agree to have it. The evidence for the specific effectiveness of ECT compared with a similar placebo procedure is persuasive (though not exactly overwhelming) and I'll discuss it shortly but by the mid-1970s, ECT had been almost outlawed in some states of the USA following pressure from anti-psychiatrists and psychiatric civil rights activists. Like many psychiatric treatments – like many medical and surgical treatments, come to that – it had sometimes been used excessively, unselectively and unnecessarily but many psychiatrists felt strongly that there was still an important place for it, especially in treating the significant minority of patients who didn't respond to the antidepressant drugs that were introduced in the 1950s, or to various sorts of psychotherapy. The trouble was that a procedure as impressive as ECT could obviously have large placebo and non-specific effects and there had been no really well-designed, controlled trials of ECT against a truly comparable placebo procedure. That would entail all patients having the anaesthetic (because that in itself is a very impressive *procedure* and thus likely to have its own non-specific effects as well as possible specific, pharmacological ones) but then randomising only half of them to the electrically-induced convulsion. To minimise bias for or against the treatment, it would have to be a typical 'double blind' randomised controlled trial (RCT) in which both treaters and treated are unaware of which treatment group patients have been randomised to. In the 1970s, I wrote several articles arguing that while ECT had been oversold and badly needed some decent RCTs, it probably did have a real, specific effect and shouldn't be banned.[58] I wrote these articles because of two patients I had treated.

The first was a 75-year-old woman. Her two-volume NHS file recorded that she had seen psychiatrists for depression almost annually for the previous 30 years; that she usually requested and received ECT; and that she always recovered quite quickly after receiving it. She began her psychiatric career in the 1930s and must have been one of the first people in Britain to receive ECT when it was introduced in 1938. Because she felt a lot better after it, she kept coming back for more. The odd thing was that she generally got better after only two or three treatments, rather than the usual half dozen. My consultant was reluctant to electrify her ageing brain again without compelling reasons, so we made a little experiment without telling her, which was easy to do then but would be unethical now. We gave her the anaesthetic but didn't push the shock button. After two 'treatments', she recovered as usual and thanked us for the nicest ECT she'd ever had. (Unlike the real thing, it didn't give her a headache.) We didn't tell her about the deception but recorded it in her case notes and hoped that it would be considered if she requested treatment again.

The second case involved a depressed Australian in his fifties. He too had previously had ECT, though only once, but he had got better after it and was keen to have another course. Though it would have been easy enough and reasonable enough to agree, I thought that his current depression had different causes compared with the first episode, when he was in his twenties. He had been successful in his profession and seemed to have no major domestic problems but he was getting a bit deaf and finding it hard to keep up with the rising stars in his organisation. I thought he should try some cognitive-behavioural (psycho)therapy first but he was adamant. Accordingly, I arranged for him to turn up to the ECT suite as an out-patient twice weekly but he only had the anaesthetic without the electricity. Although I would have started to push the shock button if he didn't improve, he got steadily better after the usual six 'treatments'. A few months later, when the improvement had been sustained, I told him what I had done because it was obviously important for him to realise that his recovery was due not to the supposedly crucial, specific and defining component of ECT but to other factors: natural resilience, spontaneous improvement and, of course, non-specific and placebo effects.

The first really big placebo-controlled trial of ECT for depression was done in Britain in 1980 by a Medical Research Council team, headed by Dr Eve Johnstone and I was present when she first presented the results at a psychiatric meeting. All patients in the trial had failed to respond to antidepressant drugs. Both groups improved considerably whether they had six real or six sham ECTs but the real ECT group improved somewhat more quickly. In other words, ECT had a real and useful effect but it also had very large non-specific effects and was nothing like as specifically effective as some of its enthusiasts had expected.[59] I was naturally pleased to have my predictions confirmed by these results, which have been more or less replicated in most subsequent controlled trials.

What I found most interesting about Eve Johnstone's presentation, though, wasn't the overall treatment outcome but the story she told about one particular patient. Mute and refusing food, he was the most depressed patient in the whole study and they had serious ethical doubts about whether it was right to give this very sick man a 50% chance of not having the real ECT that might be absolutely vital for his recovery. Fortunately, because that 'might' (or 'might not') is exactly what RCTs are supposed to clarify, the MRC team stuck to their scientific guns. Happily, the patient recovered completely. When, barely able to stand the suspense, they eventually broke the randomisation code to discover which treatment group the patients had been in, they found that this most depressed of all the patients had actually received sham ECT.

There is a comical footnote to the pro- and anti-ECT arguments that raged in the 70s and 80s. In 1975, one idea that was being mooted to improve the lot of GPs was to use nurse-practitioners to deal with most of the coughs and sneezes and other minor discomforts that still form a sizeable proportion of most GPs' workloads. This, it was argued, would be nice for the nurses, who were capable of doing much more than taking blood pressures, giving injections and dressing wounds, and nice for the GPs who would consequently have more time to deal with the more complex or puzzling cases. One of my students at Birmingham happened to mention that his father, a local GP, had employed nurse-practitioners for several years and was pleased with the results. I thought there might be an article in this, so I arranged a visit and subsequently wrote a piece about nurse-practitioners for the *Guardian*. Over lunch, the GP and I naturally talked about other aspects of medical life and he mentioned an unusual episode in his career.

At one time, he did some sessional work in a local psychiatric hospital and his duties included administering ECT. In those days, it was normal for psychiatrists to give the simple intravenous anaesthetic ourselves and then press the shock button, without involving specialist anaesthetists. The GP had little experience of ECT elsewhere but was assisted by experienced nurses. He noticed that the patients didn't seem to twitch much during the procedure but the nurses didn't mention it and he assumed that all was well. With a large dose of muscle relaxant (see below) you wouldn't expect the patients to twitch much anyway. After a year or so, a man came to do a routine service of the ECT machine. He fished out a loose lead and told them that whatever the machine was doing, it certainly hadn't been delivering any electricity to the patients. After I mentioned this story to Dr Michael O'Donnell, the editor of *World Medicine*, he asked the GP to write an article about his experiences. He agreed, provided that his identity would be protected and so, disguised as 'Dr Easton-Jones', in 1974 he wrote 'Non-ECT' which soon became *World Medicine's* most quoted article. Later, and still disguised, he was the star of a well-balanced 1983 BBC documentary on ECT in which I also took part. This happened because during planning discussions with the BBC, it emerged that the producer had been told by a Very Important Psychiatrist that the pseudonymous Dr Easton-Jones was me. I don't mind the occasional controversy but I didn't see why I should be landed with responsibility for other people's experiences, so I suggested they include the GP and let him tell his story. Predictably, both the article and Dr Easton-Jones' TV interview have been used as ammunition by opponents of ECT ever since, which wasn't what I had intended. The opponents invariably miss the point of the story, which isn't that ECT is useless, barbaric and obsolete but that the non-specific effects of impressive treatments can be amazingly powerful;

and that both doctors and patients can have unjustified faith in their specific effectiveness.

It can, of course, be argued that giving someone a general anaesthetic twice a week is not the same as giving an inert or inactive medication. That is true but nobody had argued that merely sending someone to sleep for 15 minutes, or just giving them a good night's sleep with tablets, was likely to be helpful in depression that had failed to respond to several weeks of medical and psychotherapeutic attention and anti-depressants, with or without sleeping tablets. A very recent controlled study, using an electroencephalograph (EEG) to measure the precise duration of the induced convulsions, found that longer convulsions gave significantly better results than shorter ones, though only a minority of patients recovered fully.[60] However, another paper argued that even the best-conducted RCTs of ECT are suspect because patients having real ECT are more likely than sham ECT controls to experience side effects such as headaches and memory loss (usually transient but not always[61]) and that this makes it impossible for the trials to be truly double-blind.[62]

Another reason for thinking that the non-electrical, non-pharmacological components of the whole treatment package are so important is that something similar was seen with a now-obsolete psychiatric treatment: insulin shock. The ability of insulin to cause hypoglycaemia (low blood sugar) and coma, which could easily be reversed with intravenous glucose, formed the basis of what was, from the 1930s to the 1950s, one of the standard treatments for schizophrenia in many hospitals. Unlike ECT, there was no real underlying theory but it was thought that the hypoglycaemia did something or other to the brain that was helpful in a condition that generally had a rather gloomy prognosis. It also, undoubtedly, gave psychiatrists, often resentful of their low status compared with medicine and surgery, something to *do*. Something, moreover, that was unarguably *medical.*

The procedure was labour-intensive and dramatic; serious brain damage could occur if hypoglycaemia and coma were too profound or prolonged. It lasted for an hour or two, involved repeated injections and intravenous drips and often left the patient feeling groggy for a few more hours. The doctors and nurses involved thought of themselves as a professional elite and it appears that they often selected for treatment the sort of patient who would probably have quite a good prognosis anyway. Not everyone believed that the insulin was the crucial component and in

1957, one of the earliest RCTs[63] showed that when patients and doctors were unaware of who was given insulin, there was no difference in outcome between insulin coma therapy and coma induced by a generous dose of sedatives. The elaborate ritual and the intensive nursing encouraged both doctors and patients to believe that the treatment was specifically effective but it wasn't. The apparent benefit was non-specific.

ECT is not painful, let alone 'barbaric' but to be convinced, you need to know some basic brain physiology. Originally, ECT didn't involve electricity and as every psychiatrist knows, it originated in a theory that was wrong from the start. Around 1930, a Hungarian psychiatrist called Ladislas von Meduna claimed, without providing any objective evidence, that epileptics were less likely to become schizophrenic than non-epileptics. From this unsound premise, he reasoned that epilepsy might have a protective effect against schizophrenia and so it might help schizophrenics if they could be given artificial epileptic fits. In truth, this theory was only marginally less bizarre than some of the beliefs that schizophrenics come up with because as with almost all types of brain disease or dysfunction, epilepsy can make people *more* prone to schizophrenia, not less.

Even if the error in von Meduna's thinking had been pointed out sooner than it was, the idea of inducing convulsions in schizophrenics might have been thought worth exploring. Syphilis, the AIDS of the pre-penicillin era and including brain syphilis – General Paresis of the Insane - was being treated with malaria therapy. The high fever of artificially-induced malaria could kill the delicate spirochaete bacteria that cause syphilis, so the idea of using one illness to treat another wasn't either new or absurd. Psychoses can and do clear up quickly and spontaneously but the outlook for schizophrenia that didn't improve or disappear in a few months was bad. Like kicking a faulty TV set, convulsive therapy could be defended as better than doing nothing and inactivity is unpopular with healers and patients alike.

As any epileptic will confirm, you never remember an ordinary epileptic fit. There is always a short period of retrograde amnesia, which means there's a gap in the memory from a few seconds before the fit until a variable period – usually a few minutes – after it is over. In the 1930s, it was known that giving injections of camphor or other drugs could reliably bring on convulsions and that was what they used initially. The new treatment was also tried on other unresponsive psychiatric illnesses, notably depression and the results were surprisingly impressive, as we might predict with such an impressive procedure but contrary to von Meduna's theory, it seemed to help depressives more than schizophrenics.

One big drawback was that although the drugs did produce convulsions, the convulsions took a long time to arrive. It could take up to an hour between injecting the convulsant drug and the onset of the fit. During that period, many patients experienced a build-up of very unpleasant sensations. Ordinary epileptics often experience this pre-convulsion 'aura', though it commonly lasts only a few minutes or even seconds. In 1938, concerned to minimise the discomfort of the new treatment, two Italian psychiatrists, Ugo Cerletti and Lucio Bini, hit on a solution. Cerletti had been studying experimental convulsions in animals, induced by electricity. Electricity seemed to cause instant unconsciousness in the animals but he was reluctant to try it on humans. One day, he visited an abattoir where officials had told him that pigs were killed by electricity. He expected that this would strengthen and justify his reluctance[64] but what he saw was quite different. (Squeamish or vegetarian readers may skip the next few sentences.)

To the head of the pig, the slaughterer applied electric tongs connected to the town's ordinary 125-volt supply. This produced instant unconsciousness and rigidity (the 'tonic' phase of the seizure) followed by typical 'clonic' epileptic convulsions – i.e. rhythmic spasms - but the pig's throat was cut just before the clonic phase began. The convulsions speeded up the flow of blood from the animal but Cerletti realised that it was the rapid blood-loss and not the electricity that caused death. Reassured, he and Dr Bini looked around for a suitable human guinea pig. They found one in a homeless schizophrenic, apparently without family, who had been mute for several days since his admission. (Remember: it's 1938. It is important to avoid the un-historical mistake of judging them solely by today's standards of research ethics and human rights. If you had been a doctor at that time, you would probably have done the same.) They applied the electrodes and pressed the button briefly. There was no convulsion but the previously mute patient sat up in bed and said: 'Not another one: it'll kill me'. Cerletti, perhaps murmuring the Italian equivalent of 'Trust me, I'm a doctor', pressed the button again, this time for a bit longer. It was enough to produce a convulsion and Cerletti and Bini rightly made history because they had made an apparently useful but distressing treatment much less distressing. The technique and the equipment were simple and within a few months, it was being used all over the globe. That's when CT became ECT. Cerletti himself said that he often felt "embarrassed, ill at ease and even seized with remorse" when performing ECT[65] and hoped that in time, something gentler and more dignified would replace it.

Although ECT was a great improvement on drug-induced CT, it wasn't free of adverse effects. Whether the fits were chemically or electrically induced, they could still be strong enough to cause dislodged teeth or fractures, especially in older people with soft bones. Patients were restrained to prevent them from injuring themselves on the bed during the convulsive phase, or from falling off it (hence the scene in 'Cuckoo'). The problem was solved after the war when the Amazonian arrow-poison curare and shorter-acting synthetic muscle relaxants such as scoline started to be used in anaesthesia. Curare-type drugs paralysed the muscles (including those responsible for breathing) so that much lower and safer levels of anaesthetic could be used, though artificial respiration was necessary. If ECT patients were given scoline before the electricity, the strength of the convulsions was much less and the risk of fractures or broken teeth correspondingly reduced. Sometimes, there was virtually no movement of the limbs, hence Dr Easton-Jones's lack of suspicion but as some participants in Amazonian tribal feuds presumably discovered, if there's one thing even nastier than being shot to death with arrows, it's being shot with arrows while fully conscious and sensitive to pain but progressively unable to run, move or breathe while you take ten minutes to die of bleeding and lack of oxygen. Curare and scoline paralyse but don't cause unconsciousness. (The same thing happens if you eat badly-prepared *fugu* fish in Japan.) Consequently, you have to give patients a short anaesthetic to send them to sleep before giving the scoline. Fortunately, short-acting intravenous barbiturate anaesthetics were developed around the same time. The paralysing effect of the scoline wore off before the patient regained consciousness after the anaesthetic or the fit and the whole procedure was quite simple. This 'modified' ECT was used in most civilised hospitals by the 1950s but what the 'Cuckoo' film showed was the old-fashioned unmodified version. By the 1970s, that was really a misrepresentation.

Chapter 6
Penny plain, twopence coloured
Placebo effects of medication and how to maximize them

[The explorer Wilfred Thesiger's ailing native guide] bathed in one of the hot springs, famous for their medicinal effect. The next day, Thesiger noted wryly, his leg festered with boils.
Asher M. Thesiger. A biography.

Ålesund is a Norwegian coastal town in fjord country north of Bergen. It was almost completely destroyed by a fire in 1904 and quickly rebuilt in the prevailing *Jugendstil* style of architecture (aided by Kaiser Wilhelm II, who had holidayed nearby) but one of its buildings neatly symbolises the therapeutic delusions of the time and of several preceding millennia. Among the rebuilt shops, the pharmacy was one of the largest. It is large enough to serve now as part of the town museum, yet there were barely 10,000 inhabitants in 1904 and apart from opiates, laxatives and sedatives, the number of medicines at that time with any specific as opposed to placebo effects on disease was very small. A year's supply of them for the whole town would probably have fitted comfortably into one large cupboard with room to spare. In its way, the prominence of this pharmacy in the town's architecture was as much a testimony to faith as the pyramids of ancient Mexico, the temples of Angkor Wat or the great cathedrals of Europe. The prayers for the sick that were uttered in Ålesund's numerous churches also lacked specific effects but as with the act of taking medicines, the act of praying often helped those involved to feel better and – with some important qualifications to be discussed shortly - almost regardless of the contents of the medicine bottle or the prayer.

In 1904, nearly all of the medicines given to sick patients had no beneficial effect on the natural course of the diseases from which they suffered and only placebo effects on most of the symptoms of those diseases. Often, they caused damage to healthy organs and that damage was sometimes lethal. This ineffectiveness applied whether the medicines were prescribed by qualified doctors, by folk healers or by homoeopaths, though at least the homoeopathic medicines had no toxic effects, since they had no true organ-modifying effects at all. One of the very few exceptions to this litany of ineffectiveness, the use of citrus fruit juices to prevent or cure scurvy, involved a fruit, or eating a normal, balanced diet rather than a medicine and long predated the discovery of vitamins and deficiency diseases.

Morphine was good for relieving pain, cough and diarrhoea. A standard pharmacology textbook of 1905 acknowledged that 'Opium', from which morphine is derived, '[is] the most important article of the whole *materia medica*'[66] but opium didn't *cure* anything and at that time, you could buy opiates in many countries without a prescription and even from a grocery. If you were already vulnerable because of illness or age, brisk diarrhoea might finish you off and therefore opium might occasionally make a life-saving difference. If you got cholera and experienced the massive diarrhoea, dehydration, electrolyte loss and kidney failure that killed the vigorous 53-year-old Tchaikovsky during an epidemic in St Petersburg, opium would be unlikely to save you. I expect his doctors gave Tchaikovsky plenty of it but what he really needed was an intravenous drip containing sodium and potassium salts and glucose, all of which were available at the time. Glucose was first identified and isolated in the 18th century. *Fin de siècle* St Petersburg was home to several internationally famous medical researchers but his failure to receive these simple chemicals just shows how little even the best physicians of the time understood about what is now basic physiology and pathology.

A little booklet titled 'Principal Drugs and Their Uses', written by 'A Pharmacist' and undated but, judging from the phraseology and illustrations, probably also published around 1900, contained hardly any drugs that were effective, let alone curative.

Quinine still prevented or aborted most types of malaria in an era before drug-resistant parasites had evolved.

Thyroid extract reversed the effects of hypothyroidism.

Even before vitamins were discovered in the 1920s, cod liver oil, rich in Vitamin D, was apparently used for rickets as well as other things but only after the damage from poor diets and too little exposure to sunlight had been done.

A few vaccines appeared late in the 19th century following the earlier and serendipitous discovery of smallpox vaccination but tetanus antiserum and vaccine were not discovered in time to prevent thousands of agonising deaths from tetanic spasms from infected penetrating wounds in the First World War.

Digitalis, from the common foxglove, helped some types of heart disease and the swollen legs that went with it; but that's about all.

The list is short and unimpressive. By 1905 chloral, paraldehyde and various barbiturates were available for poor sleepers. Ether, nitrous oxide and chloroform were used for general anaesthesia and cocaine for nerve blocks. (Cocaine's stimulant effects and over-the-counter availability had already caused the first epidemic of non-traditional drug abuse in the Western world.) The demand for laxatives, popular with both doctors and patients in a bowel-obsessed culture but rarely necessary for health and sometimes dangerous, was also well catered for.

A 1904 price list for the most important drugs of the time manufactured by the leading British pharmaceutical company, Burroughs Wellcome, contains only about 40 distinct classes of chemical, very few of which had any curative value. Most had no specific therapeutic effects of any kind and several were actively harmful without being helpful. Yet the price-list has an illustration of Burroughs Wellcome's vast factory in open country east of London, the manufacturing equivalent of Ålesund's grand pharmacy and Angkor Wat. Its largely useless products provided the capital that Henry Wellcome bequeathed to the nation to create the admirable Wellcome Trust for medical research and its museum and library.[67] Hypertension (high blood pressure) is a common cause of strokes and heart disease but as late as 1945, President Roosevelt died, aged 63, of a stroke that might have been prevented if effective antihypertensive drugs had existed.

Apart from the ineffectiveness of most of its products, there is one other important difference between the pharmaceutical industry then and now. In 1905, most of its drugs were manufactured in response to demand from the doctors who prescribed them. Other than Bayer's aspirin – a synthetic version of a traditional remedy and used in those days purely as a mild pain-killer – the pharmaceutical industry had hardly started to do the research and development that within a decade or two would give us the first of a long list of 'magic bullets' with real and often powerful effects. The flip side is that instead of being essentially the servant of the medical profession, the industry (and its shareholders) has increasingly become medicine's master. Particularly in psychiatry, this means that it not only manufactures drugs but also manufactures diseases (and associated scare stories) for its drugs to treat. The classification of bereavement as a 'disease', for example, was seriously put forward by some psychiatrists.

In populations where poverty, dirt, poor health and malnutrition were rife, as the British army discovered to its surprise when conscription was introduced in 1916, giving patients clean surroundings and decent food for a change might make the difference between recovering from wounds or chronic illness and not recovering. They wouldn't make much difference in acute illnesses like pneumonia that could kill you in a few days, before the improved diet, fresh air and warm bed could have any restorative effect. The medicines had no curative properties mainly because even the best-educated doctors knew very little about the chemical and physiological processes that went on in the various organs. They knew what all the organs looked like and they knew what most of them did, in a general way, but as to how they did it, not much was known.

Type 1 diabetes is a common illness that used to be almost invariably fatal. The pancreas had long been familiar as an organ but the discovery that it was involved in blood sugar control was only made around 1900. It was another 20 years before insulin was identified as the main pancreatic hormone that did the controlling. Two years later, large-scale production of insulin from slaughtered animals ended the distressing sight of diabetic wards full of dying children and adolescents. (How many strictly anti-vivisectionist or vegan diabetics, I wonder, made a hypocritical exception for insulin?)[68] Apart from very low-carbohydrate diets introduced just before the discovery of insulin that had their own hazards, *nothing* that was given to or done to diabetics before insulin appeared had any effect on the basic disease process. Two-thirds of patients under ten usually died within a year or two of diagnosis[69] but as with almost all illnesses, some spontaneous recoveries or milder disease variants occurred. If prayers had been said and saints invoked, such recoveries would be called 'miracles'. The English language, in all its marvellous richness, lacks an equally specific word to describe what happens when prayers and saints fail to avert a fatal outcome.

Although it did not require an understanding of the physiology of any known organ, there were advances on the anti-bacterial front, once the concept of specific infections with specific bacteria had been experimentally demonstrated and confirmed. Antiseptics and aseptic technique made surgery much safer and allowed surgeons to be steadily more adventurous but the treatment of infections (as opposed to their prevention) was not a success story of the 19th century. Despite the appearance of few effective serums and vaccines for bacterial and viral infections, the many people who continued to die from acute and chronic infections included surgeons who pricked or cut themselves while operating on infected patients. Unlucky or careless surgeons continued to die from this cause until sulphonamides appeared in the 1930s and penicillin in the 1940s. These days, the main risk to surgeons seems to be Hepatitis C. A brilliant medical school contemporary of mine died after the disease progressed to cirrhosis and liver cancer.

Any follower of the priapic adventures of Dr Samuel Johnson's biographer James Boswell knows that mercury was the standard treatment for syphilis until the 20th century. ('A night of Venus, a lifetime of Mercury' as Boswell's contemporaries joked.) Syphilis probably arrived in Europe with Columbus and its skin lesions had several new features that marked them out from other skin disorders, though misdiagnosis was probably common. Sufferers were treated with mercury, usually absorbed through the skin after repeated rubbing with mercury ointment. Patients soon experienced acute side effects, after which the rubbing was stopped or interrupted but mercury also has long-term side effects. Teeth often fell out. After receiving mercury treatment, the 18th century diarist William Hickey described how "my tongue and mouth became so inflamed that I could take no other nourishment than liquids". Mercury treatment almost certainly had no specific effect on the disease and even if it had, any small benefits would likely have been heavily outweighed by its sometimes lethal toxicity. When industrial mercury waste was discharged into Minamata Bay in southern Japan, contaminated seafood caused catastrophic neurological damage to both the living and the unborn, pets as well as humans.

A problem with measuring the effects of any treatment for syphilis, especially before RCTs, is that like many other diseases, syphilis has a very long and variable course. Some people only get the primary sore, usually on a sexually exposed area (which can include surprising and unexpected places). It disappears spontaneously in a few weeks and may never progress to the secondary stage – typically a highly infectious generalised rash – or the more dangerous tertiary stage, when bones and internal organs, as well as the skin, are affected. These organs include the brain and brain syphilis accounted for up to a third of all admissions to the asylums for the insane that were established in most Western countries in the 19th century. It was familiar enough for Ibsen to make it a major theme of one of his best plays – 'Ghosts'. (Presumably it wasn't just the syphilis that got it banned for so many years but even more taboo themes like incest and euthanasia.) Some patients had tertiary syphilis without any secondary manifestations but the tertiary stage usually occurred many years after the initial infection and was by no means always fatal. In the infamous Tuskegee Syphilis Experiment, in which African-Americans with syphilis were deliberately left untreated even after penicillin became available, more syphilitic patients died than in the treated and no longer infected control group but not vastly more. Only an RCT lasting many years could have shown whether mercury was any good and lengthy trials are difficult enough to organise and complete even now. As with blood-letting, mercury treatment was popular with both patients and doctors despite the harm it caused, presumably because both were impressive procedures and had some impressive immediate side effects. You can easily see the similarity with impressive, demanding and popular religious rituals. Another recent controlled trial found that a placebo nasal spray, wrongly believed by the experimental subjects to contain a powerful opiate painkiller, reduced experimental pain more if it contained a peppery substance that irritated the nose.[70] "Our results revealed that nasal sprays with a side effect lead to lower pain than inert nasal sprays without side effects. The influence of side effects on pain was dependent on *individual beliefs* about how side effects are related to treatment outcome, as well as on expectations about received treatment." [my italics]

Apart from that small handful of drugs that could actually prevent, reverse or ameliorate serious disease (early vaccines, thyroid extract, quinine, digitalis for heart failure) almost nothing from the extensive pharmacopoeia of pre-1920s medicine favourably affected the natural course of most illnesses, especially life-threatening ones. Colchicine, extracted from the autumn crocus, relieved the excruciating pain of acute gout and is still sometimes used but it didn't stop the uric acid crystals caused by gout from eventually silting up the kidneys and causing death or invalidism from kidney failure or hypertension, as well as wrecking their joints. Since doctors didn't know *how* colchicine or digitalis worked but only that they seemed helpful, they were unable to develop better versions of them by tweaking their mechanisms.

Another small handful of treatments included drugs and other interventions that may have been genuinely helpful but only for conditions that were not very serious. My favourite of these may be apocryphal but has the ring of truth about it. One technique for treating nocturnal enuresis – bedwetting – involves an electrical sensor that detects wetness and immediately wakes the patient, thus helping to retrain the bladder and its brain connections. A traditional West African precursor of the enuresis alarm involved tying a particular type of frog to the child's leg. This amphibian was silent in dry conditions but noisy in wet ones. Enuresis brought forth loud croaks that woke the child. Conversely, the fact that the common dandelion is called *'pis-en-lit'* (piss-in-bed) in France probably denotes a true diuretic (i.e. urine-promoting) effect. Diuretics can be useful in hypertension and some types of heart disease but for them to be useful, the diseases first need to be identified and at least partly understood. Blood pressure couldn't be easily measured until the early 19th century. The relation between kidney damage and hypertension wasn't discovered until a century later. There is no evidence that dandelion leaves were specifically recommended for conditions that might have responded to them.

Doctors don't like to feel powerless in the face of disease, especially serious, disabling and life-threatening disease and patients don't like to think that their doctors are powerless. These two very understandable viewpoints explain why, despite the lack of effective drugs, doctors prescribed, and patients swallowed, pills, tablets, capsules and liquid medicines with great enthusiasm. Both doctors and patients often felt better, though in different ways, after all this prescribing and swallowing and both doctors and patients often believed that the fact of feeling better was causally related to the pills, tablets etc. that had so enthusiastically (or in some cases, anxiously and reluctantly) been swallowed. They were both nearly always wrong, yet there were many grateful patients like Gerald and many doctors like Sir Bentley, whom we met in the Introduction, who got genuine pleasure, as well as status and a good income if they treated prosperous patients, from feeling that they had contributed usefully to the sum of human happiness. When a visitor to an art exhibition told the painter Claude Monet; "I don't know much about art, Monsieur Monet, but I know what I like", Monet is said to have replied; "Yes Madame. So do the cows". Like Monet's cows, the average patient doesn't know much about medicine but she too knows what she likes.

We all tend to feel better after taking things called 'medicines', in part because we hope, expect and want to feel better. If we believe ourselves to be seriously ill, that hope and want may be quite desperate. The Bible tells us that we should 'honour the physician' but even if it didn't, sick people will always call for someone to take away that terrible pain in their stomach or chest, stop them from feeling they're about to suffocate, restore their vision or make their paralysed legs move again. And, of course, to take away the ultimate über-fear that they may soon be dead. Whether the person who answers the call is a doctor or some other sort of healer, they are expected and programmed to *do something*. The "physicians of the utmost fame", in Hilaire Belloc's *Cautionary Tale of Henry King,* who simply turned up, took one look at Henry and then "answered as they took their fees/There is no cure for this disease" were, to put it mildly, atypical.

Many diseases improve or disappear without treatment and Darwinian natural selection often ensures that some people survive or avoid diseases that kill most of those affected, as happened in the 2015 epidemic of ebola fever in West Africa. Before effective treatment became available around 1995, some people never developed AIDS despite being infected with HIV for many years. *Homo sapiens* and most other living things both animal and vegetable would hardly have survived if resistant strains did not exist or evolve. Unfortunately, like the man in the elephant joke, doctors have often believed that they had healing powers that they did not, in truth, possess. They still do, though in conventional medicine, scepticism and therapeutic humility are much commoner than they used to be. The same cannot be said for Complementary and Alternative Medicine where scepticism is generally unwelcome, as it is in most religions, especially where the sacred texts are concerned. Although new plants (and thus new herbal medicines) are always being discovered or analysed, most herbal medicines of today would still be familiar to the herbal medicine prescribers of the 18th century, many of whom were physicians. Conventional doctors have stopped using most of them because they did not appear to be effective, or were less effective than newer or purer compounds but CAM practitioners continue to use them. It is in this context that any claims for the objective or purely subjective benefits of religion must be considered and evaluated, for religious rituals have also not changed much in the last several hundred years and it is probable that no really new ones have appeared.

One really crucial factor or 'variable' in the size of the placebo effect is what one may call the sales technique of the prescriber (who often, in the world of CAM, is literally a salesman). The practical importance of this point cannot be overstated because it is clear that placebo and non-specific effects in medicine and religion can be increased in ways that are simply not possible with specific pharmacological or surgical interventions. If I give you antibiotics for pulmonary tuberculosis due to a strain of the TB bacillus that is sensitive to those drugs, the infection will nearly always disappear if it isn't so far advanced that it kills you before they have had time to take effect. It may take several months but it will disappear and the difference in outcome between antibiotic and placebo is not just statistically significant but massively, obviously and clinically significant as well. Provided the antibiotics are taken as directed, not only will the infection disappear but any anatomical damage done by the TB bacillus to lungs or joints will, at the very least, not progress further. In the placebo group, although some spontaneous recoveries will occur, many patients will suffer further damage and some will die of the disease, often because of haemorrhage from a lung artery whose wall is breached by adjacent tubercular infection, as happened to the poet John.

If I have given you the right doses, then increasing the dose will not speed your recovery and may delay it because of increased side-effects. I cannot directly increase the real and demonstrable bacteria-killing ability of those antibiotics by being very positive and reassuring, spending more time with you, wearing what you regard as the right sort of clothes for a proper doctor, telling you how lucky you are to be treated with a wonderful new drug, giving you additional but inert injections or impressively coloured tablets, or any of the several other non-specific things that collectively constitute the placebo effect. If you were a noted unbeliever and if I happened to know, say, Richard Dawkins, I could arrange for him to drop by and leave you a signed copy of his latest book. If you were a noted Catholic, I could ask the local bishop to bring a few holy relics and say a few prayers in place of the Dawkinsian equivalents. I could ask the medical school's music society or jazz club to send some musicians to your room. None of these things would directly increase the specific effects of the antibiotics but any or all of them might well improve your mood and morale. That in turn might have useful, though entirely non-specific, effects on your ability to overcome the infection by, for example, better cooperation with chest physiotherapy or a more positive attitude that may even affect your immune system and stimulate your body's natural defences. (In animals, as we shall see, immune system activity can be significantly altered for better or worse depending on the way in which they are handled.) The negative and equally non-specific effects of reducing morale and expectations can be seen in the previously-mentioned 'Hound of the Baskervilles' effect among Chinese- and Japanese-Americans but not White Americans. Their increase in mortality from chronic heart disease was 15% on the unlucky fourth day of the month and no other explanation satisfactorily fits the facts.[71]

An important corollary of this is that in contrast, it is very easy indeed to increase the size of the non-specific effects and their religious equivalents by tweaking any of the components just listed, to which many others could be added. Up to a point, the more of them that I provide and the more impressively I present them, then the greater may be the improvement in your morale. The famous and unusually sceptical 17th century English physician Thomas Sydenham understood that potential very clearly, writing: "The arrival of a good clown exercises a more beneficial influence upon the health of a town than of twenty asses laden with drugs". His hunch that most medicines of his time were not only useless but toxic as well ("I confidently affirm that the greater part of those who are supposed to have died of gout, have died of the medicine rather than the disease") adds to his greatness. A recently published Catholic manual on exorcisms shows that the Vatican understands that potential too. The instructions for handling an "emergency case of grave oppression and possession" include (as well as the usual props such as "exorcised salt, a crucifix, a relic of a saint, a manual of deliverance prayers") advice to wear the right sort of clothes ("a purple stole"), to "place one hand on the forehead of the afflicted person (with the relic cupped within your palm)" and to say everything using "a commanding and firm tone".[72] This is not a book published long ago by some fringe Catholic body or eccentric cleric. It has the approval of the author's archbishop Dr. Gaudencio Rosales. "After examining it thoroughly in the light of the established norms and policies of the Archdiocese of Manila, we hereby grant the Imprimatur, declaring it free of error in matters of faith and morals". In Italy, the town of Isernia apparently boasts five exorcists – one of them a bishop - for its population of 60,000 souls.[73] In Rome itself, a Vatican-affiliated university, the spendidly-named Regina Apostolorum Pontifical Athenaeum, regularly "held a semester course for priests who want to become exorcists".[74] I mention the practical details not to mock or dismiss exorcism, which may sometimes, in my view, be an appropriate procedure for a devout person whose belief that she is possessed does not stem from schizophrenia but to show how similar are the mechanisms underlying both exorcism and placebo effects. More on that later.

Another important corollary is that where randomised controlled trials show the effectiveness of a particular drug to be only marginally better than the placebo control (even if the difference is technically within the limits of statistical significance) it is possible that by using a different sort of placebo control, especially if individualised to be more impressively in tune with some of the patient's beliefs and preconceptions, a practitioner skilled in the black arts of placebo psychology and non-specific mechanisms might get consistently better results with the placebo than more scrupulous or less enthusiastic doctors might get by using the 'active' drug. This is especially relevant to drugs used in psychiatry, where differences between active and placebo medication in RCTs are quite often small, where placebo factors are particularly important and powerful and where there are often numerous negative RCTs to set against the positive one. For example, in one trial, two groups of psychiatric patients were randomised to receive a sedative or a placebo. Group 1 had no other treatment and two weeks later, about a third – 35% – of them had improved whether they received active or placebo medication. Group 2 had the same drugs but also a day of intensive psychological testing that involved elaborate machines, flashing lights and a placebo injection. Two weeks later, about 70% of both active and placebo patients reported improvement.[75] Antidepressants are often prescribed for the treatment of anxiety as well as depression. In a study of the widely used antidepressant escitalopram for social anxiety, one group of patients received the drug overtly while in the other group, the same dose was given covertly in the guise of an active placebo. Three times as many patients (50% vs 14%) responded in the overt group and their improvement was twice as large.[76]

In some RCTs of medicines, 'blinding' of patients, researchers or both may be difficult to achieve or maintain and this conscious or even sub-conscious 'unblinding' could bias the outcome of the trial in either direction. Drugs with noticeable side-effects may reveal themselves to observant nurses and doctors as well as to patients. Where this is a problem, the use of an 'active placebo' may restore blinding. Active placebos contain a drug that causes mild side effects – such as a dry mouth – that mimic the main side effects of the real medication but the drug is thought not to have any therapeutic (or anti-therapeutic) effect. The similarity of side effects makes it difficult for both patients and doctors to discover inadvertently which group the patients are in: drug or placebo. The results of such trials typically show smaller differences between the two groups than those obtained by less rigorous methodology but active placebo controls are used in only a tiny percentage of RCTs.[77] An alternative technique for preserving blinding, or cancelling out the effect of unblinding, is the 'crossover' design, in which the patients exchange groups half-way through the trial or at some other point. In one celebrated trial that would probably not be administratively or ethically approved today, the head researcher, a psychiatrist, announced that the crossover would take place six weeks into the trial. The nurses and psychologists who were monitoring and assessing the patients duly noted changes in the rating of various symptoms six weeks later, because they thought they had been able to identify at least some patients as being in one group or the other and therefore reported not just the changes they observed but also the changes they consciously or unconsciously *expected* to observe when the crossover happened. The psychiatrist, however, had cunningly cancelled the crossover. The patients remained on the same medication or placebo throughout the trial, but the staff doing the rating rated them as they expected they would improve or worsen when they took or discontinued what the staff hoped would be an effective drug. This 'Heaton-Ward effect' is named after the sceptical and constructively devious psychiatrist who deceived his colleagues as well as his patients in the higher interests of scientific and therapeutic truth.[78]

In 2015, a series of papers appeared in *World Psychiatry*, the usually unexciting journal of the World Psychiatric Association, sent free to tens of thousands of psychiatrists world-wide. The theme was the small differences in effectiveness between placebo and active drug in most antidepressant trials. The final paper of the series – 'What if placebo effect explained all the activity of depression treatments?'[79] – begins: "Many randomised trials have shown that when depressed patients receive no active treatment, e.g. they are administered pill placebo, a large part of them improve anyway ... The corollary is that many patients remit even when undergoing exotic therapies such as Argentinian tango, swimming with dolphins or horticulture". Another paper discusses the curious finding that the small differences between active and placebo depression treatments may have been getting even smaller in the last decade or two. A large recent US survey found that the 3-fold differences between states in suicide rates were not explainable by the more than 3-fold differences in antidepressant prescribing but were persuasively explained by the even larger differences in gun ownership and firearm suicide.[80]

Since the pharmaceutical industry as a whole tries hard to suppress negative studies because they are bad for business, that makes the potential power of placebo effects correspondingly easier to overlook and allows dishonesty to flourish. A typical example was uncovered in 2015 by a team dedicated to "restoring invisible and abandoned trials" (RIAT).[81] Despite the evasiveness or indifference of most of the leading participants in the original study, the RIAT team were able to discover several undeclared institutional, financial and perhaps even ideological conflicts of interest and serious irregularities in the statistical analysis of the results. The authors turned a study of an antidepressant which had essentially negative findings into a paper that was used to promote the widespread use of a drug that had at most a marginal and questionable value. However, just as important as the pharmaceutical researchers' dishonesty and self-deception is the fact that they were revealed by medical academics with classic sceptical scientific attitudes. (The incidental discovery that supplies of placebo medication in this trial were compromised at one point because the placebo had passed its expiry date deserves a place in some future anthology of surreal or anti-bureaucratic jokes.) At least medicine, unlike religion, sometimes questions its positive claims.

Research into placebo effects as specific phenomena rather than as incidental findings in RCTs is a recent but growing field. SIPS, the Society for Interdisciplinary Placebo Studies was only founded in 2010 and held its first conference in 2015. Among several interesting findings is that even when patients are given a medication that they are *told* is a placebo – what is called an 'open-label placebo' – they can still experience significant beneficial placebo effects.[82,83] This had been noticed in another study from the 1960s, in which some psychiatric out-patients improved so much that they refused to believe that the tablets really were inert placebos, assumed they were a new and wonderful drug and demanded repeat prescriptions.[84] Its rediscovery means that some of the ethical objections to using placebos in treatment or research can be overcome. The important implications are discussed in detail in the final chapter.

Chapter 7
Birds do it, bees do it
Placebo and non-specific effects in animals and babies

If placebo effects work mainly through belief, expectation, suggestion, sales-talk, hope and faith, how can non-human animals also experience them? With the possible exception of 'expectation' – since creatures ranging from fish to dogs pick up cues that indicate the imminence of feeding time – animals seem unlikely to have these emotions and cognitions except in rather rudimentary forms, if that. Jeffrey Masson, who appears later in the book as a critic of psychoanalysis but is mentioned here for his subsequent interest in animal rights, reports that among academics who study animal behaviour and animal psychology, animals are not supposed to have any human-like emotions at all. [85] "Animal behaviourists, zoologists, and ethologists have been fearful of being accused of anthropomorphism, a form of scientific blasphemy ... Not only are the emotions of animals not a respectable field of study, the words of emotion are not to be applied to them".

Even if we share Masson's belief, as I think I do, that on this point of principle, the academics may be wrong, that does not, in my view, mean that animals and humans have similar concepts and understandings of disease, medicines, prognosis, recovery or death. Especially death. Yet controlled trials, exactly the same sort of RCTs that we have already discussed in human patients, show that animals, like humans, can be profoundly affected by the non-pharmacological components of therapeutic interventions: by placebo and non-specific effects. This is easily explained if we shift our focus for a while from 'placebo' and return to the second component of that phrase: 'non-specific effects'. Human patients generally feel better after a consultation, especially if augmented by a physical examination and blood tests, scans and other impressive and sometimes uncomfortable procedures that have no overt therapeutic function at all. Sceptics may respond that while humans generally know that people in white coats or bearing other outward and visible signs of their medical status are associated with relief and usually have good intentions, animals have no such prior knowledge. That is probably true, especially for animals that have had no previous contact with a veterinary surgeon or clinic. Animals may not know the intentions or capabilities of the humans who handle them in therapeutic or research settings but the effects of handling are apparent not just in immediate changes in heart-rate or respiration but also in processes that can affect recovery from disease, such as the immune system. Placebo effects in human surgery are "related to the patients' expectation and the 'meaning of surgery', whereas the non-specific effects are caused by fluctuations in symptoms, the clinical course of the disease, regression to the mean, report bias, and consequences of taking part in the trial, *including interaction with the surgeons, nurses, and medical staff*".[86] (my italics) In a veterinary setting, that 'interaction' is largely the handling that animals get.

A review of placebo effects in animals[87] from which the following quotations are taken notes that "animals have been the main subjects in experimental studies of the mechanisms of the placebo effect for over 70 years". Yet despite the enormous growth of veterinary medicine for both food animals and pets, "To the author's knowledge, studies specifically examining the placebo effect in therapeutic trials have not been reported. ...Most importantly, in trials in which the placebo is selected as the control method,[88] *untreated groups that serve as second controls to distinguish placebo effects from other causes of disease resolution are not used*". (emphasis mine) Bear that in mind the next time a homoeopath or acupuncturist insists that their treatments can't be 'just placebos' (as if placebo effects were something trivial) because animals, as well as humans, respond to them. And bear it in mind the next time a vet recommends expensive drugs for your ailing dog or cat, especially if the problem is behavioural rather than due to infection or other obviously physical disorders. The increase in prescribing of antidepressants and anti-anxiety drugs for pets is as worrying, and as questionable, as it is in humans.

One important non-pharmacological mechanism in animals is simple Pavlovian conditioning. It is so powerful that animals can be trained to respond to drugs in ways that are the opposite of their pharmacological effects. Pavlov[89] himself noted that after dogs were given repeated doses of morphine in an experimental chamber, morphine-like effects were detected as soon as they were put into the chamber and before they received any morphine. When rats were repeatedly injected with scopolamine, a sedative that had consistent and predictable effects on their ability to learn new tasks, similar effects were seen after an inert, placebo injection of saline. In another dog experiment, repeated injections of morphine were given at doses that caused vomiting and sleep. After ten days, saline injections produced the same responses but after a few more days, "the same physical response was elicited merely by the arrival of the experimenter in the room". Remarkably, even some of the powerful behavioural and physiological effects of large doses of insulin could be replicated, after Pavlovian conditioning, by a saline injection.

Even more important, from a therapeutic point of view, than these relatively simple direct and immediate results of Pavlovian conditioning are the longer-term effects that conditioning and non-specific mechanisms can have on the immune system. "In rats, pairing the neutral stimulus of a sweet taste (saccharin) with the immunosuppressive drug cyclophosphamide [eventually] resulted in an immunosuppressive response to saccharin alone". This may have important implications for the treatment of some very serious diseases, including systemic lupus erythematosus (SLE) – the auto-immune disease which, within a few days, struck down the Labour leader Hugh Gaitskell in 1963 at the age of only 56.[90] In mice specially bred to be genetically susceptible to the disease, "development of SLE, as measured by age of onset, [protein in the urine] and mortality was dramatically delayed by conditioned immunosuppression, compared with non-conditioned animals, *thus offering definitive evidence that a pharmacologically inactive conditioned stimulus – a placebo treatment – can have a substantial and positive therapeutic influence on the course and outcome of a disease state in animals"*. (emphasis mine) One researcher concluded that "all neutral cues *(places, persons, things, procedures and rituals)* surrounding the specific medical therapy may be classically conditioned by association with previously experienced ameliorative effects that have occurred in these environmental settings". (My italics) This is really important stuff and has obvious implications for both medicine and religion, though as many excited researchers and journalists have discovered to their annoyance and disappointment, what seems to work for animals doesn't necessarily work for humans, or even has the opposite effects.

Equally remarkable are studies that show the powerful effects of various ways of handling animals. As any anxious parent of a sick child knows, the immediate effects of being handled by doctors and nurses can be bad as well as good, especially if white coats are associated with having needles stuck into you or with painful changes of wound dressings. Those bad effects – not placebo but *nocebo* – get a more detailed discussion later but both sorts of response affect animals as well. "In rats undergoing [thyroid surgery], mortality rate was 13% in a group petted and handled gently by a human each day since infancy, as compared with 79% in a group not handled and petted". When rabbits were fed a cholesterol-rich diet, the resulting arterial changes were less than half as severe if they were held and petted several times a day compared with the control group. However, many other studies indicate that "human contact increases stress in animals" and that stress can also cause immunosuppression. In animals with cancer, the same immunosuppression that was so helpful in treating SLE can cause an increase in the growth of tumours that might otherwise be inhibited by the immune system. That would certainly count as a nocebo effect.

There may be no animal studies that compare placebo medicines with *no* treatment (i.e. with spontaneous improvement or recovery) as well as comparing active with placebo medicines, but there are, as with humans, several trials that show only small advantages, or no advantage, for pain-relieving drugs compared with placebo. Like ageing humans, dogs too become arthritic, or need orthopaedic surgery. RCTs of carprofen, an ibuprofen-like drug, showed that it was better than placebo for canine arthritis but when it was used for post-operative pain, 8 of 10 dogs given carprofen needed at least one dose of morphine in addition, compared with only 5 of 9 dogs in the placebo group and the carprofen dogs needed more morphine than the placebo dogs.[91] The apparent superiority of the placebo is not statistically significant (i.e. it could be due to chance or inappropriate methodology) and I would not draw too many conclusions from the study, except that perhaps vets, too, tend to overestimate the specific effectiveness of commonly used drugs and to underestimate their placebo and non-specific effects. And that it is important that results from clinical trials be independently replicated, preferably more than once, before anyone gets too partisan about a treatment - for or against.

Like animals, very young children cannot tell us clearly and directly how they feel and they too are presumably not influenced by anything specific by way of 'belief, expectation, suggestion, credulity, hope and faith'. The same lack of more than the most basic beliefs, expectations and so forth probably applies to people with severe congenital learning disability as well. As adults, many of them cannot tell us much more than animals and babies can about how they feel but like babies and animals, people with severe learning disability (IQ between 20 and 65) demonstrate placebo and nocebo effects.[92] If they also develop Alzheimer-type dementia, as happens frequently in Down syndrome, placebo effects disappear, as they do in severely demented adults. Perhaps the demented can still respond, up to a point, to such important non-specific factors as interaction with other humans (or animals) and to 'handling'.

Another thing that children, adults with severe learning disability and animals have in common is that assessments of any changes following placebo or active interventions have to be made by third parties. Not only are the patients unable to tell us in any detail how they feel but it is also impossible to measure changes in muscle strength or mobility, for example, by asking them to move a limb in a particular direction or to try as hard as possible to lift a weight, as one would normally do. This reliance on indirect information brings us to another under-researched but important aspect of placebo effects: the phenomenon of *placebo effect by proxy*. As one of the very few papers to discuss it notes, "...people other than the patient may also feel better when a patient receives placebo treatment". They "may have an emotional response to a patient's treatment and think that the treatment is helping the patient even in the absence of any direct physiological benefit to the patient or indication from the patient that the treatment is working".[93] One important group of those 'other' people who often feel better when a placebo has been administered are the CAM practitioners who think they are providing a specifically effective treatment that, in reality, has no specific effects. Spiritual and religious 'healing', whether formal or incidental, may also be sincerely perceived when in reality it has not happened. Religion, which so often embodies and promotes hope, may be a dangerously fertile soil for this kind of error. Conventional doctors are certainly not immune to it but their professional education should at least give them some incentive to be on guard. From the moment they enter medical school, they learn about the importance of randomized controlled trials; and the more rigorous, transparent and free from conflicts of interest, the better.

In an economic sense, the most important group who wrongly perceive benefit may be the patient's family members. "Parents of a child with a viral upper respiratory illness may believe that the child needs antibiotics, and parental expectations or the doctor's perception of parental expectations (or both) may influence prescribing patterns. Antibiotics are overprescribed in these situations and function as 'impure' placebos: the psychological benefit to the parent, such as a relief from worry, represents placebo by proxy."

My Melbourne experience bears that out. Media-led demands for health services to fund essentially placebo treatments are not uncommon. (See Ch. 14) Such campaigns can simply be dishonest or due to journalists ignorant of the null hypothesis – that the effect does not exist – but desperation for a good story by victims of JDHD

(Journalist Deficit Hyperactivity Disorder) usually reflect hope that is unsupported by sound evidence. We can forgive this misplaced faith among patients and their anxious friends and relations, though in the medium and longer term we should also try to improve their awareness of the facts that honest and methodologically sound research tries to provide. We should perhaps be less forgiving when misplaced faith and hope affect and motivate the people who provide the treatment, especially if they have strong financial or emotional interests in one particular intervention and even more especially if it is the main or only treatment that they happen to provide.

Chapter 8
Wise men from the east
Acupuncture and Traditional Chinese Medicine

Hardly a month goes by without an excitable medical journalist telling us about a herb used in Traditional Chinese Medicine (TCM) that is a promising or even sure-fire treatment for some currently fashionable scourge of Western lifestyles. A brief Wikipedia search might have made them pause before inflicting their enthusiasm on us. The carefully recorded dates of birth and death of successive Chinese emperors during lengthy periods of history reveal that despite all those herbs, many of the emperors died young. During the Ming dynasty, established in AD 1368, nine of the first 13 emperors never made it beyond 40 and all but one or two of them died from diseases rather than violence. Long before that, in 210 BC, China's first emperor, Qin Shi Huang, who commissioned the famous terracotta army, launched an obsessive search for the elixir of life before dying at 49.[94]

The throne passed to most Chinese emperors when they had already reached or neared adulthood and had therefore survived or avoided the considerable medical hazards of infancy and childhood. In neighbouring Tibet, whose inhabitants seems to be regarded by some TCM enthusiasts as being even more in touch with sources of ancient oriental wisdom than the Chinese, they did things differently. After 1483, Dalai Lamas were identified and chosen when they were still children, though well past the particularly dangerous first year or two of life and then reared at court in the capital, Lhasa. Although they presumably had a better diet and better access to traditional Tibetan medicine than the average, dirt-poor Tibetan subsistence farmer, several infant Dalai Lamas died before reaching adulthood. Of the first ten Dalai Lamas chosen in childhood during the period corresponding with the early Ming emperors, three died before reaching 20 and another three before reaching 30. Of the remaining four, the oldest only made it to 67. It is difficult to avoid concluding that ancient Tibetan and Chinese medical wisdom, even with added acupuncture, was just as ineffective at preventing and treating life-threatening illness as its ancient occidental equivalents. Eventually, as in other countries, Chinese and Tibetan standards of living improved and Chairman Mao's 'barefoot doctors' brought some benefits of science and basic Western medicines to the benighted peasants, as well as better hygiene. In the long run, their efforts possibly made up for the millions of lives lost during Mao's man-made famines and his colonial war in Tibet.

Acupuncture is a more familiar example of Ancient Oriental Wisdom.[95] The Chinese, one argument runs, have been around for a very long time and look as if they might soon run the planet. 1.4 billion of them can't be wrong. Acupuncture's specific and defining doctrine is that some sort of undetectable, unmeasurable, indefinable but healing *energy* courses through the body along channels called 'meridians'. It supposedly has powerful regulatory effects on many organs and tweaking it by sticking needles into special points along the meridians can affect those organs in ways that benefit health. It is an older variant of the vitalism that became popular in Europe in the 18th century and gave us Mesmerism and homoeopathy. One thing that should immediately make us doubt this claim is that the list of organs includes some, like the meridians themselves and the 'triple stomach warmer', whose existence has not been noticed or confirmed by several generations of increasingly skilled Western anatomists. Acupuncturists who believe in meridians thus have to insist that even if science cannot detect them, or the *yin, yang* and *chi* that supposedly run through them, they are nevertheless there in some mysterious way, although we cannot see them. As with several other CAM doctrines, this is very similar to the Christian doctrine of transubstantiation.

Unlike homoeopathy or psychoanalysis (soon to be discussed) acupuncture did not have a named and messianic founding guru. It apparently began as a fairly culture-specific folk-remedy in ancient China and neighbouring lands, much as the trephining of skulls was a particular (though not exclusive) feature of pre-Columbian Andean and Meso-American civilisations. The Chinese kingdom continued to develop and is still with us under different management. So is acupuncture, though in China itself, acupuncture has been in and out of fashion at various times in the past few hundred years. Chairman Mao initially derided it, then promoted it, though his personal physician claimed that Mao never used acupuncture or other traditional Chinese medicines himself. I once visited a modern 4000-bed Chinese hospital in Chengdu that had a department for TCM and acupuncture. My hosts said that its main function was as a kind of *oubliette* for patients with ill-defined complaints who had not responded to conventional treatments. (The hospital also had a large English-Chinese notice board bearing the names and locations of the various departments. Among facilities with unremarkable English descriptions such as x-ray, gynaecology, allergies, surgery and psychiatry, I spotted one that described its departmental function as 'cunt examination'.)

Acupuncture first intruded into Western consciousness in a big way during the thaw in US-China relations towards the end of the Viet-Nam war. When President Nixon visited China in 1972, acupuncture was among the things that the visiting Americans were shown. In particular, they saw patients allegedly having thoracic or even cardiac surgery entirely under acupuncture anaesthesia. According to some reports, patients were said to be clutching Chairman Mao's Little Red Book and singing his praises as the surgeons made their incisions. I was a junior anaesthetist for a while but you don't need to be an anaesthetist to realise that that was very unlikely to be true. When the thorax is opened, the lung on that side collapses. Cardiac surgery usually means opening both sides of the thorax and patients would die very quickly from lack of oxygen unless they were intubated and had air pumped into their lungs. This requires an endotracheal tube to be inserted through the larynx and Nature and evolution have very sensibly arranged that if even small objects get into your trachea, you cough very vigorously until they are expelled. Inserting an endotracheal tube cannot be done without very heavy sedation or lots of local anaesthesia. You can't sing Mao's praises when a tube is separating your vocal cords but when observers are disposed by personality, political ideology or circumstances to be credulous, impressionable and enthusiastic, they do not always make reliable observations. Religious healers and their audiences have the same problem. However, given adequate oxygenation, even thoracic surgery can sometimes be done under local or hypnotic anaesthesia.

Acupuncture is claimed to be good for many very different illnesses. Even in supposedly scientific journals, the list of conditions or symptoms that allegedly benefit *specifically* from acupuncture includes pain, stroke, pregnancy, asthma, irritable bowel syndrome, depression, alcohol or opiate withdrawal, nausea, fatigue, insomnia and cancer. When therapeutic enthusiasts tell you that their favoured treatment is good for almost everything, you can be confident that it's time to smile politely and move away. A personal reason for scepticism about acupuncture was the claim made by a Harley Street acupuncturist who gave a talk to our student medical society. After telling us that appendicitis could be confidently diagnosed just by taking the pulse in a special Chinese way, he said in response to a question about sterilizing acupuncture needles that it wasn't necessary. The needles, he told us, were made of gold and gold was a 'self-sterilising' metal. That was questionable even in 1962, before the danger of getting hepatitis from shared needles was appreciated.[96] Solid gold is not 'self-sterilising' and by the 1970s, epidemics of viral hepatitis caused by insanitary acupuncturists were being reported. There were also cases of pneumothorax (collapsed lungs) after needles inserted by anatomically ignorant acupuncturists penetrated into the thoracic cavity.

As I hope you realise by now, a major obstacle to increasing objectivity and reducing bias in RCTs of acupuncture is the difficulty of comparing the real thing with a sham placebo procedure that cannot easily be identified as a sham. This requires ingenuity but if it can be done with surgery and ECT, it ought to be possible with acupuncture; and it is. This is shown by the surprising results of a unique study that debriefed selected patients after they had a good response to what they did not realise was sham acupuncture.

Prof. Ted Kaptchuk is one of the increasing number of academics doing research into placebo effects with a view to incorporating them deliberately into medical practice. He was also one of the pioneers of placebo research, following a period in China studying acupuncture and Traditional Chinese Medicine. One of his team's most revealing studies has very important implications for treatment in general and its religious equivalents. It involved patients in the placebo wing of an RCT of acupuncture who had improved.[97] As the authors explain; "Although participants give informed consent to be randomized to verum [i.e. true, active drug] or placebo, they are typically never told which treatment they actually received: they are not debriefed to treatment allocation". In this unique study, Team Kaptchuk debriefed them. They also went to a lot of trouble to ensure that the placebo procedure felt so much like acupuncture to the patients that they could not easily tell it from the real, skin-penetrating thing. "Well-designed placebos resemble the real (verum) treatment in every possible way.... Design features such as visual appearance, taste, and smell, make the [ideal] placebo indistinguishable from verum treatment. If trial participants can reliably distinguish between placebo and verum treatments and thus identify their treatment, then blinding is considered to have failed *and the trial's validity is questionable.*" [my italics]

In trials of acupuncture, it is particularly important that the simulated placebo procedure be as difficult as possible to distinguish from the real, 'active' or 'verum' procedure. Given the nature of acupuncture, it is also quite challenging but because acupuncture is a popular CAM treatment for which many claims are made by both practitioners and patients, several ingenious solutions to the challenge have been devised. In some ways, they resemble the war-winning tactics of the people who spent much of WW2 devising ways of misleading the Nazis by making them think that things were not happening when they actually were (e.g. preparations for the D-day landings) or that things were happening when in reality, they were not (e.g. feeding false information that caused more V1 flying bombs to explode south of London in open countryside).

Kaptchuk and his team had done a placebo-controlled trial of acupuncture in irritable bowel syndrome (IBS)[98] a common condition with no clear cause (or with a range of possible causes) that often does not respond well to conventional medical treatment and thus understandably leads many unhappy and dissatisfied sufferers to consider CAM instead, or as well. Patients were randomly allocated to one of three wings: a waiting list 'no treatment' control, placebo acupuncture with deliberately brief and limited therapist-patient discussion, and placebo acupuncture with an initial 'augmented' 45-minute discussion to "develop rapport". Kaptchuk later described the augmented consultation as 'at least 20 minutes of ... "very schmaltzy" care ("I'm so glad to meet you"; "I know how difficult this is for you"; "This treatment has excellent results"). Practitioners were also required to touch the hands or shoulders of members of the [augmented] group and spend at least 20 seconds lost in thoughtful silence'. It could equally be described as sales-talk. The placebo needle, validated against the real thing in previous studies, touched but did not penetrate the skin, retracting instead into the handle. The trial lasted six weeks and after the first three, patients were re-randomised either to continue placebo acupuncture or to switch to real acupuncture. 262 patients took part, a group large enough to provide some statistically robust data. As an incentive to persevere, participants were told they could have further real acupuncture without charge after the study ended.

The first finding, and this far into the book I hope, not surprising, is that "As hypothesized, 'augmented' consultations resulted in clinically and statistically significant improvements beyond those resulting from limited consultations". In other words, patients who received - or perceived themselves as receiving - a lot of attention, however scripted and insincere,[99] did better than patients who received much less attention. This is an important but entirely non-specific effect. Progress was assessed at three and six weeks and from the whole treatment group, a small number were selected for 'debriefing' about their allocation to placebo or active groups. Of those who had improved – and this is the unique feature of the study - an even smaller number, three men and one woman, were given the opportunity for an extended discussion of their experiences of the treatment and of their responses when they learned that they had received placebo acupuncture for the whole six-week period.

The aim was "to elucidate the meaning of the phenomenon for a particular person in the context of their lived and felt experience. To achieve this elucidation, the researcher must put aside presuppositions and enter the lifeworld of the participant through a bracketing process. This involves setting aside personal and academic assumptions about the phenomenon (internal suppositions) as well as other wider assumptions connected to the external phenomenon (external suppositions) for the duration of the analytic process". In other words, this was not an exercise in medical or investigative elitism. It was a genuine attempt to enter into the patients' worlds in order to learn something useful from their thoughts; something, furthermore, that might help doctors and patients to make better use of placebo and non-specific effects that in this study, as in so many others, were considerable. Unlike many medical papers, this one often quotes the patients' own words and the fact that "To our knowledge, no such descriptions have been reported previously" adds to its importance.

Before the debriefing, 'Frances' described how "She found acupuncture relaxing and as she went through the trial her symptoms improved and she experienced very little abdominal pain and reduced bloating". Her attitude to acupuncture – her faith in it, if you prefer – was positive even before she started it. "I'm a firm believer in acupuncture. My mom did and a few other people I know have had it and they've always had positive results from it. So you know, I figure, hey, any kind of acupuncture is bound to make a difference in something. I don't know exactly what. Maybe they're sticking needles where there is nothing". Frances was surprised when she learned that she had been in the all-placebo group because she was sure that she had felt the needles go in; ("mine went in deep").

'Alan' "believed that he had real acupuncture. He based this on noticing his acupuncturist's actions and his associated sensations, and thought that he could feel the acupuncturist pushing some of the needles in deeper than others. During one treatment he fell asleep and was woken up by a needle poking his wrist, which again suggested to him that he was receiving real acupuncture. Alan also experienced effects on his IBS symptoms (mainly reduced gas) and an increased sense of calmness." He too was "surprised to find out he had placebo. He questioned this, he questioned the news that the placebo needle does not pierce the skin, and he questioned whether his acupuncturist was indeed an acupuncturist. He then worked up a positive interpretation of his being on placebo, *that it shows how important mental factors are in IBS.*" (my italics)

'David' "described how his acupuncturist changed the points that she used during treatment and he interpreted this as meaning that she cared for him and was giving him real acupuncture. His IBS symptoms and overall well-being improved which he partly attributed to 'an emotional thing' (consistent with his identity as 'an emotional person') and he thought that his feeling emotionally supported by the 'wonderful' study personnel was enhancing the acupuncture's effects. By the end of the study, he felt so connected to and cared for by his acupuncturist that he could not imagine her giving him placebo." He too insisted that the placebo needles had definitely pierced his skin. "I always thought I was so relaxed, I would fall asleep. It was just like wonderful. Uh, so, emotionally, part of the whole thing, the thing is that - even though you call me the placebo group, I don't consider it totally placebo group because there are other benefits that came out of it that would not have happened if I'd not been in this study. So it may be placebo and I accept that, but there were other things that I know made me feel better because I was in this study."

'Ben' had a "belief in alternative medicines in general" but had previously had a good response to medication. He too was surprised to learn that his skin had not been pierced. Like most participants, he saw the study as a way of helping humanity and IBS sufferers in particular, as well as something that might relieve his own IBS symptoms. Like Alan, he rationalised his positive placebo response ("he was calmer, had a whole new outlook, and his symptoms improved") as one facet of an acceptance that IBS had "a lot to do with the mind" – a view with which many of those who treat it would agree. He also seemed to understand one of the main components of placebo responses. "But it gives me, it tells me something good about myself, that, you know, if I want to be healed, I could be healed."

Another finding of this and other studies by Team Kaptchuck reinforces an important point that I have made several times, precisely because it is so important. It is that *symbolism, meaning and setting* can be crucial in determining the nature and size of placebo (and nocebo) responses and that each of them is a very individual or even idiosyncratic phenomenon. "These four participants' experiences each have unique features and the particular setting (an acupuncture trial) must be remembered." In another paper, they write: "Placebo effects are often considered the effects of an inert substance, but that characterization is misleading. In a broad sense, placebo effects are improvements in patients' symptoms that are *attributable to their participation in the therapeutic encounter, with its rituals, symbols, and interactions.*"[100][my italics] For 'therapeutic', read 'religious' as well. There are obvious similarities between patients who feel definite physical sensations (as well as the relief of symptoms) after contact with pseudo-needles, and people who feel similar changes after contact with pseudo-relics and pseudo-prayers. One extremely important feature of Kaptchuk's trial of pseudo-acupuncture was that the recipients really were blinded to the true nature of the procedure. They could not distinguish between the real thing and a convincing facsimile and in both cases, the supposedly crucial importance of the defining features of the intervention – needles and penetration for acupuncture, holiness (however defined) for the relics, prayers and water – were shown to be *of no importance at all.* In both cases, the changes – large or small, good or bad – were entirely typical of placebo, nocebo and non-specific effects.

Kaptchuk's team are not the only people studying realistic placebo acupuncture in IBS and several sham techniques have been studied that seem equally effective in deceiving recipients.[101] An even more recent study also concluded: "The lack of differences in symptom outcomes between sham and true treatment acupuncture suggests that acupuncture does not have a specific treatment effect in IBS".[102]

Chapter 9
Pies in the sky
Placebos in war, weather, gastronomy, sport and politics

We must realize that the default mode of human psychology is to grab onto comforting beliefs for purely emotional reasons, and then justify those beliefs to ourselves with post-hoc rationalizations.

Steven Novella. Skeptics' guide to the universe.

If *homo sapiens* found relief from present anxiety and reassurance about the future in religious beliefs and activities when facing only the ordinary hazards of existence, it is easy to understand why warriors facing even higher and more immediate risks of injury and death are so attracted to the placebo effects of religion and other comforting rituals. They also incline to the 'heads-I-win-tails-you-lose' argument, praising their preferred deity when they defeat their enemies but blaming themselves (or occasionally, the Devil) when they don't. Since most history is written by the victors, there are more accounts of successful wars, supposedly aided by appeals to the winning side's deity, than of defeats that occurred despite earnest prayers to the god of the losers. As Sir John Squires' wrote in 1916:

> God heard the embattled nations sing and shout
> "Gott strafe England" and "God save the King!"
> God this, God that, and God the other thing –
> "Good God!" said God, "I've got my work cut out!"

The Roman Catholic church is particularly keen on selective evidence for divine favours. In Malta, the church of Sta. Maria Assunta in Mosta proudly displays a 250kg bomb that crashed through its impressive dome (the third-largest in Europe) during an air-raid in April 1942. It failed to explode, as many unsophisticated bombs do, a fact that happily saved the Royal Navy from even greater and possibly crippling losses during the Falklands War with Argentina in 1982. In any case, a similar 'miracle' saved Conway Hall in 1941 during the London blitz, even though it was built for and occupied by the thoroughly God-rejecting South Place Ethical Society.

The claim that 'there are no atheists in foxholes' means no more than that soldiers often resort to comforting rituals during or before battles. Military historian Anthony Beevor records that as the Soviet army advanced on Berlin in 1945, "Many soldiers kept [the words of a popular Russian song] in their left breast pocket and read it silently to themselves like a prayer in the moments before they went into the attack"[103] There are many accounts of soldiers who carried a Bible in their breast pocket which absorbed the shock of a bullet but Bibles are not the only life-saving agents. During the Spanish Civil War, a volunteer in the left-wing International Brigade took with him a copy of Marx's *Capital* in the hope of mastering its complex arguments. One day, he was shot in the chest but - thanks be to Marx - he only suffered bruising, commenting later that "not even a bloody bullet could get through that book". Beevor also reports that one evening, "in what amounted to a mass secular baptism, 2000 Red Army soldiers...were received into the Communist Party". Meanwhile, on the Nazi side of the lines, Himmler in an Order of the Day claimed that "The Lord God has never forsaken our people and he has always helped the brave in their hour of greatest need." As Beevor remarks, "Both historically and theologically, this was an extremely dubious assertion".

Most prayer in time of war is an individual, informal, unorganised activity unsuited to randomised controlled trials, especially in the heat of battle but it can be studied retrospectively by anthropologists. In Israel, where both anthropologists and, regrettably, wars are plentiful, it has been possible to study at least the incidence of prayer among different sorts of people exposed to war and some of the effects of prayer on their behaviour and mood. In 2006, Richard Sosis, an anthropologist attached to an American university, happened to be in the country when Hezbollah fired several thousand rockets from Lebanon into northern Israel, causing great alarm among the civilian population. Those who did not simply move temporarily to less vulnerable areas devised a range of responses to the bombardment, of which reciting psalms from the Old Testament was the most popular, especially in the northern town of Safed which was home to an ancient community of rabbinical scholars and students as well as the largely unbelieving and non-observant citizens who are more typical of Israelis.

For psalm-reciters who were actively religious, the procedure reduced their anxiety levels, like familiar rituals of any kind, but it did not make them less likely to take sensible precautions. In contrast, the nominally unbelieving Israelis who recited psalms took fewer precautions subsequently. They *felt* safer but actually exposed themselves to more risks.[104] That is a variety of *nocebo* effect – a harmful or undesired effect due to a placebo. For a particularly impressive military example, we need to take ourselves back to RAF Bomber Command's strategy of bombing Germany into submission. Flying to and from German cities in large, slow and unmanoeuvrable planes was a dangerous business, even at night. Losses of around 10% on each mission were not uncommon and Bomber Command lost more of its members, about 60%, than any other large unit of the British armed forces. Aircrews had to deal with night-fighters over enemy territory and with anti-aircraft guns and searchlights over the target cities. Being caught in the concentrated beams of several searchlights must have added considerably to their feelings of vulnerability. Individual aircrew often took with them 'lucky charms'. Others persuaded themselves that they were being flown by a 'lucky' pilot who had survived for longer than the average but just as both patients and doctors may come to believe that a particular intervention is curing, relieving or preventing certain illnesses when it actually makes matters worse, so may the military – both those in the front line and those who send them into battle – develop a misplaced and damaging faith in particular bits of military hardware.

By this, I don't mean the ordinary jingoistic beliefs that 'our' guns, planes, tanks and ships (and men) are better than 'theirs'. Prof R V Jones, one of the main players in Britain's very successful intelligence war against the Nazis, described how "Bombers were frequently being caught in German searchlights, and the idea had grown up that searchlight control could be upset if the bomber switched on its IFF (Identification Friend or Foe) radar recognition set, and so the bomber could then escape. The proffered explanation was that the searchlights were directed by radar, which was somehow jammed by the British IFF".[105] Jones pointed out to the RAF that there was no evidence for any protective effect. There had been no campaign from above to persuade aircrew to use their IFF in this way. It was an evidence-free belief – a superstition – that had simply spread among the aircrew; what we might now call an airborne myth. However, as Jones warned, there was an obvious risk that the Germans might pick up the radio waves emitted by the IFF device and use them to detect and intercept the bombers. Bomber Command reluctantly agreed to investigate Jones' fears. They claimed to find no positive evidence one way or another but "argued that it was a good thing that pilots go on using IFF because it will encourage them to press home attacks against defended areas when they might otherwise be inclined to turn tail." Even a year later, they said that "It is known...that many crews think the device effective and it should therefore be retained ... Since no evidence has come to light indicating the harmful effects [of leaving on IFF] the psychological effect on the crew alone is sufficient to justify its retention".[106] This response is similar to the one often used by some CAM defenders and their religious equivalents who say that if a treatment makes people feel better, then it is effective and shouldn't be criticised.

If the Germans didn't realise that they could use IFF emissions to locate and destroy British bombers in 1941, when Jones first warned the RAF, they had certainly done so within a year or two. Jones reported: "It appears inescapable that IFF has betrayed some of our bombers. Legends about the effect of IFF on searchlights may now be reaping a tragic harvest and future tragedies of similar type will only be avoided by the peremptory application of common sense to shatter quasi-scientific superstition".[107] By 1944, intercepted German messages confirmed that IFF transmissions accounted for a significant proportion of successful interceptions. As soon as the RAF and the US Air Force accepted this and sharply restricted the use of IFF and other radio-emitting devices, losses diminished considerably.

The RAF crews only deceived themselves and had no financial or fraudulent motives. Unfortunately, throughout history, placebos and fraud have often been linked – a sad but important fact that should be kept in mind when evaluating claims for effectiveness. A much more recent case involved the military use of a device that had only placebo effects but its use over several years added significantly to the still-growing number of deaths from car-bombs in Iraq. The ADE651 was supposed to be able to detect explosives and was bought in large numbers by the government, who spent over £50 million on them. Investigations as early as 2001 showed a precursor of the device to be useless, merely a glorified dowsing rod[108]. The ADE651 itself was exposed in 2008 as a scam by journalists and by the military of more sceptical countries but Iraq bought 1500 of them in that year and the following one. It turned out that one of the ministers involved had been bribed by the manufacturers but reporters interviewed several Iraqi soldiers and policemen who insisted the device was effective. They included Major-General al-Jabiri of the Interior Ministry's General Directorate for Combating Explosives.[109] The device was even exhibited at an arms fair in 2009 but although it was sold for up to $60,000 per unit, the cost of its component parts was cents rather than dollars. The manufacturer eventually received a long prison sentence but in the world of fraudulent cures, that sort of justice is unusual. These three examples neatly illustrate the way that placebo effects in medicine and elsewhere make people persist in doing things that are unhelpful and may be harmful, when they could be thinking and behaving in more constructive ways.

Similar placebo effects and misplaced faith can still be seen in another kind of conflict – the perpetual war against insects and small mammals that bite us, damage and pollute our dwellings and occasionally cause disease. For the apparently increasing number of people who think that the mammals have at least as much right to exist as we do and who draw the line at killing them, electronic devices that claim simply to make the creatures flee from ultrasonic or electromagnetic emanations are understandably popular. The manufacturers may honestly believe they are effective but do they have any specific effect? Does it matter, in other words, whether or not the devices actually emit the sound-waves or electromagnetism that are supposed to be the specifically active component of the intervention? Apparently not, according to the International Association of Certified Home Inspectors[110], who cite numerous academic studies and note rather tellingly that although "Cats and dogs can hear in the ultrasonic range, ... they appear not to be bothered by the noise emitted by these devices. ... Nevertheless, many users have reported success".

Guns are not only used to kill people or animals. They can be fired in salutes or as reinforcements to the percussion section in performances of Tchaikovsky's '1812' overture. They can even be used to try to alter the weather. In the dying years of the Austro-Hungarian Empire, an Austrian wine-maker was regularly worried by the possibility that autumnal hailstorms might ruin his grapes just as they were getting ready for harvesting. Rain was good but hail was bad and you could never tell when the former would turn into the latter. The vine-grower in question was called Herr Siegel and he had an Idea. Maybe, if you fired shrapnel from a cannon into suspect clouds, any lurking embryonic hailstones would obligingly change from ice to water and save his crop.

It happened that the first time he made this experimental intervention, the clouds above his own village disgorged rain while those above several neighbouring villages poured hail onto the trembling vines and their unhappy owners. The word got round. Soon, the local valleys echoed to the thunder of ever-larger rain-cannons. Like any impressive placebo, the noise was reassuring and satisfying but the results of objective study were not. When some sceptic (or perhaps a believer honestly seeking confirmation of his belief) got round to a careful regional tally of hailstorms, rainstorms and the discharges of the various rain-making blunderbusses, the guns were found to have had no effect. However, as late as 2021, "Mysterious booms shaking the small town of Hammonton in New Jersey in December were traced to a backyard attempt at cloudbusting. Construction worker Rob Butkowski built a device resembling a giant horn to fire shockwaves into the sky, aiming to prevent hail damaging his vines... Butkowski believes it is highly effective. 'You can see the split clouds apart,' he told his local newspaper. 'You can hear it rip'."[111]

Few people who take their food seriously would be surprised to learn that the taste of food and wine is affected by how they are served. Details as large as the overall ambience of a restaurant or dining-room, or as small as the appearance and weight of the glasses, plates and cutlery, can affect taste or enjoyment. Even supposedly expert wine-tasters can be misled by disguising or falsifying the price and origin of the wine, a misperception presumably related to their expectations and thus having much in common with the therapeutic misperceptions and expectations that are an important aspect of placebo effects in medicine. Symbolism can affect both perception and expectation and a study of the effects of different types of music on wine tasting[112] found that "ratings of the taste of the wine reflected the emotional connotations of the background music played while they drank it. These results indicate that the *symbolic function* of auditory stimuli (in this case music) may influence perception in other modalities (in this case gustation)". [emphasis mine] If symbolic and emotional connotations can change the experience of wine-tasting, it's hardly surprising that they can also change the experience of pain, anxiety, fatigue, nausea and other sensations that have a large psychological element. Whatever causes such symptoms, they are among the commonest reasons why people consult healers in the first place.

For athletes, maximising the amount of blood that flows through their muscles is fundamental for success and the focus of much of the cheating and doping that blights modern sport. Glucose is muscle's basic fuel but simply increasing blood glucose is unhelpful because the limiting factor in burning up glucose is not the glucose supply but the oxygen supply. Blood oxygen is mainly stored in the haemoglobin component of red blood cells (erythrocytes) and there are several banned techniques for raising erythrocyte levels in addition to the permitted but not very effective one of training at high altitudes, where reduced atmospheric pressure may slightly stimulate the body to increase red cell production. The main banned methods are concealed transfusions of blood, either the athlete's own that has been stored for a few weeks (thus giving the body time to replace what has been taken) or blood from a compatible donor. This method was used by the disgraced US cyclist Lance Armstrong. The transfused blood may also be concentrated so that it contains an increased proportion of oxygen-carrying erythrocytes. The other method is to use erythropoietin, a hormone that stimulates erythrocyte production. It follows from this that anything done or taken by an athlete before a competition that reduces the number of erythrocytes will, in principle, reduce peak muscle performance.

Yet one of the news stories of the 2016 Rio Olympics involved the much-decorated US swimmer Michael Phelps, whose torso showed the characteristic circular bruises of a procedure called 'cupping'. He was not the only athlete to have had this permitted and very ancient 'treatment'[113] which is a current fad in CAM. It's not surprising that cupping isn't banned in athletics because its only possible effect on the oxygen-carrying capacity of the blood would be to reduce it very slightly. Cupping, like using leeches, used to be an alternative to blood-letting in the days when removing large quantities of blood from patients was believed to be helpful in many conditions. Instead of bleeding (cutting into a superficial vein and letting the blood flow) cupping involved creating a vacuum in a small cup, usually by burning something inside it to expel the air, or by an air-pump. When applied to the skin, the vacuum caused a small area of bruising or even a blood blister in exactly the same way that a love bite does. If erythrocytes are thus permanently moved from the circulation into the skin, they obviously cannot carry oxygen to the muscles.

The amount involved is very small compared with the normal blood volume of around 5 litres. In purely physiological terms, it probably made a negligible difference and Phelps's medal-winning record is apparently due in part to the fact that he has a mild form of Marfan Syndrome, which gives him longer limbs than someone of similar weight and aquatic drag. Given the trouble athletes take to get literally every last drop of blood to where it matters, it might seem an illogical choice of performance-booster but logic is not always important in choosing a placebo and that is how cupping should be seen in this or any other context. Like praying before a match, having a pep-talk from the coach or wearing a lucky charm, cupping might make performers feel more confident and even perform marginally better in an activity where small margins matter but the mechanisms are purely placebo and non-specific.

Probably without realising its similarities to the worries about illness that contribute to placebo effects, *Guardian* journalist Jonathan Freedland noted that during the public mood of fear and anxiety following the March 2016 Islamist bombing in Brussels,[114] "people are, understandably, desperate to believe there is something that can be done. For this is what is so disabling about terror: the fear that it might be entirely beyond our control. ... So people are bound to grab hold of anything that promises – however falsely – to put control back in their hands". Freedland was deploring the way in which some people put their faith in political interventions of which he disapproved, such as "exiting the EU, sacrificing their civil liberties, or even turning on a single religious minority". He may be right that such responses demonstrate the "classic...liberal mistake of thinking rational evidence can best[sic] what is, in fact, emotional and visceral" but the history of religion and medicine shows the importance of the "emotional and visceral" in human affairs and both wise doctors and wise politicians do not ignore it, even if they privately deplore it. Emotional and visceral factors are at the heart of placebo and non-specific effects and "people are, understandably, desperate to believe there is something that can be done", especially when reminded of their mortality. That is why I expect placebo effects, religion and CAM to persist. Murderous conflicts have been the norm throughout recorded history and Islamist attacks are just one of their latest manifestations.

Another aspect of placebo effects that might usefully be borne in mind by both the politicians who confidently promote new 'solutions' to real or perceived problems and the people who elect them is the null hypothesis. If the RCT is notoriously the rock on which many a new and brightly-painted therapeutic ship has been wrecked, the null hypothesis advises us to be permanently unsurprised when yet another shipwreck occurs. Enoch Powell's rueful observation that "all political lives...end in failure" often applies to political policies as well. As in medicine, many interventions by governments have no specific effect or make the problem even worse. Any changes that do take place are often random fluctuations or due to factors unrelated to the new policy but as with CAM and religion, improvements are invariably credited to the policy and its underlying theory (and the politician) while changes for the worse are either ignored or blamed on the patient (i.e. the public) for not taking their political medicine in the right way. Finally, because politicians, as well as CAM and the pharmaceutical industry, have a habit of massaging, falsifying or 'disappearing' data to satisfy their ideological or financial agendas, it is the job of transparent and incorruptible academics (the Edzard Ernsts, Ted Kaptchuks, Ben Goldacres and Archie Cochranes in the case of medicine) to record the shipwrecks and draw attention to them.

Chapter 10
Smile, please
The negative effects of positive thinking

In her famous essay on Hollywood, Pauline Kael described it as a place where you could die of encouragement.

Christopher Hitchens. Vanity Fair 'Tumortown' Nov 2010

She was a woman who did not attend Mass and who had buried her husband in a civil ceremony; according to her pupils, she hadn't even been baptized, which seemed not so much scandalous as unbelievable, like saying someone had been born with the tail of a fish. As this person's conduct was irreproachable, the Viscountess hated her all the more: 'because', she explained to the Viscount, 'if she drank or had lovers, you could understand her lack of religion but just imagine, Amaury, the confusion that can be caused in peoples' minds when they see virtue practised by people who are not religious'.

Irene Nemirovsky. Suite Française

Amy Claire is a London-based blogger who wrote a rather good article[115] about the unspecified but evidently chronic illness from which she suffers and the attitudes to this illness held by many of her fellow-sufferers:

> "The vast majority of people with my medical condition are religious, as evidenced by messages on the internet support group of which I am a member. There are hundreds of members, and messages with religious content are a daily occurrence. Often, sufferers require surgery – when this happens, emails whip round asking for 'surgery prayers'. When an operation is successful, god[sic] gets part or all of the credit: on one occasion, a woman wrote that she knew the surgeons had done their bit, but the *real* reason she survived and benefited from the surgery was that god had been watching over her.

> Of course, when things go wrong, it's a pretty safe bet that god doesn't get the blame. As though the deity were a favourite child who can do no wrong, there is no end to people's willingness to let god off the hook. When someone dies of the condition (deaths are thankfully rare), god is praised for taking them up to heaven to be with him. When surgery fails to help a person and they continue to suffer, again god is thanked and praised for not making things any worse. When things do get worse, it is presumed that god has a mysterious reason for allowing this, and the prayers continue to be solicited, the thanks still given. One woman wrote thanking god that she could hear the children playing outside while she was ill in bed; presumably it didn't occur to her to blame god for the fact she was bed-bound in the first place. And so it goes."

Not all religious people let their deity off the hook in this way. Many lose their faith when they can no longer reconcile the existence of bad things with belief in a world designed by a benevolent deity. Often, disillusionment comes late in life, when a spouse or grandchild dies in a particularly painful and degrading way, though sometimes a single subjectively or objectively shocking demonstration of the nastiness of life and the randomness of death is not enough. One of the rabbis interviewed in the clergy survey discussed in Chapter 3 said that his faith could cope with the Holocaust because that was man-made but he lost it after seeing a film of a lion chasing and eating a zebra. (That seems a bizarre conclusion to me but as with placebo effects, different folks need different strokes.)

Ronald Franz was a US serviceman and "a devout Christian" whose faith was not seriously damaged even after his wife and only son – a medical student – were killed by a drunk driver in Okinawa, where he was stationed. Once he had recovered from this calamity, his Christianity was presumably one of the things that led him to take indigent Okinawan boys and girls under his wing and put two of them through medical school. In his 80s, he encountered a gentle but earnest and naive idealist called Alex McCandless who wanted to try living in the wilderness. Franz's protective and Christian instincts were re-kindled. "When Alex left for Alaska, I prayed. I asked God to keep his finger on the shoulder of that one. I told him that boy was special. But he let Alex die". Alex died, probably from inadvertent plant poisoning and starvation, in an abandoned bus, miles from the nearest habitation in the middle of Alaska. "When I learned what happened, I renounced the Lord. I withdrew my church membership and became an atheist. I decided I couldn't believe in a God who would let something that terrible happen to a boy like Alex".[116]

In 'Smile or Die', her amusing and well-referenced critique of what may be a particularly American tendency to encourage 'positive thinking'[117] (though perhaps Americans just write about it more often) the columnist and writer Barbara Ehrenreich describes how a diagnosis of breast cancer gave her an unexpected entrée into this curious mirror-world where a positive spin not merely can but must be put on every feature of the disease and its treatment. As she puts it rather neatly, it is not simply a question of calling a glass half-full rather than half-empty. It is a question of "exhortations...to see the glass half-full even when it lies shattered on the floor". Positive thinking is widely held to be good not only for the mood of the patient but also for combating the cancer itself. Since Ehrenreich used to be a cell biologist, her ability to read and understand the scientific literature on breast cancer and on the alleged life-enhancing and death-postponing benefits of positive thinking is better than that of many women. Superficially, it might seem an attractive idea that positive thinking can kill cancer cells and even if it doesn't, surely it's a Good Thing in itself? Sadly, as Ehrenreich relates, there are several arguments against it.

Firstly, despite early reports of clinical benefit in a number of illnesses, the weight of scientific (as opposed to ideological) literature seems now to be at best equivocal and there is persuasive evidence that positive thinking can have negative effects. For example, positive thinkers are more inclined to take risks, rather like the psalm-reciting Israelis encountered earlier. Ehrenreich extends her review to cover economic as well as medical effects and few will dismiss her suggestion that positive thinking had a lot to do with the excessive optimism and lack of reality in financial circles which led to the 2008 banking crisis that started in the US and the global recession that followed it.

Secondly, even prominent exponents of positive thinking, such as the psychologist Marvin Seligman, admit that it comes "at a cost perhaps of less realism". He could say the same about most religious dogma.

Thirdly, she quotes the distinguished US surgeon, medical writer and 2014 BBC Reith Lecturer Atul Gawande as noting that "Whether one is fighting a cancer [or] an insurgency...the key, it seems to me, is actually negative thinking: looking for, and sometimes expecting, failure".[118]

Finally, she notes that the culture of optimism makes it difficult for people to reveal and discuss their true feelings and thus to deal with their legitimate concerns. It also fosters feelings, in those who are not doing well, that lack of progress or relapse are somehow their own fault for not being positive enough. (Something called 'The Just World Hypothesis' encourages this kind of blame-the-victim attitude.)[119] Perhaps we should not be surprised that it was an American associate editor of *American Psychologist* – the journal of the American Psychological Association – whose eagerly adopted theory about a simple mathematical formula for happiness was demolished a few years ago.[120] (It was a 'critical minimum positivity ratio' of precisely 2.9013.) Perhaps significantly, the demolition-squad included that very European sceptic and serial debunker Prof. Alan Sokal, whose celebrated spoof paper 'Transgressing the Boundaries: Towards a Transformative Hermeneutics of Quantum Gravity', submitted to the post-modernist journal *Social Text,* was published unaltered by them even though it was littered with deliberate and far from subtle absurdities. The journal then refused to publish a follow-up letter from the authors exposing the hoax and discussing its implications, thus ensuring that both the article and their attempt to censor criticism of it became widely known.[121]

After commenting in a breast cancer support website about "the debilitating effects of chemotherapy, recalcitrant insurance companies and" - perhaps unwisely - "sappy pink ribbons", Ehrenreich received mostly "a chorus of rebukes". One respondent told her she needed to "run, not walk, to some counselling". The only person to agree with her was someone in the terminal stages of breast cancer, who complained about "all the smiling faces of survivors, who make it sound like it is OK to have breast cancer. IT IS NOT OK". Ironically, this terminal response was posted under the heading 'What does it mean to be a breast cancer survivor?'. Hitler's propaganda minister, Goebbels, was an accomplished positive thinker. In the last few months of the war, his diaries manage a positive spin as the allies closed in unstoppably from east and west, even though they were presumably written mainly for his own benefit and not as part of his job to preserve Nazi morale. Ehrenreich notes that ex-president George W. Bush was similarly – and disastrously - afflicted with optimism, quoting Condoleeza Rice, his secretary of state for foreign affairs, who reported that "she failed to express some of her worries [about the 2003 invasion of Iraq] because 'the president almost demanded optimism. He didn't like hand-wringing, pessimism or doubt'." In an article headed 'What I heard about Iraq', the distinguished US writer Eliot Weinberger reported; "I heard the vice president say that the war would be over in 'weeks rather than months'. I heard Donald Rumsfeld say: 'It could last six days, six weeks. I doubt six months.'...I heard the vice president say: 'The Middle East expert Professor Fouad Ajami predicts that after liberation the streets in Basra and Baghdad are "sure to erupt in joy". Extremists in the region would have to rethink their strategy of jihad. Moderates throughout the region would take heart. And our ability to advance the Israeli-Palestinian peace process would be enhanced.' I heard the vice president say: 'I really do believe we will be greeted as liberators.'...I heard that the president said to the television evangelist Pat Robertson: 'Oh, no, we're not going to have any casualties.' I heard the president say that he had not consulted his father about the coming war: 'You know he is the wrong father to appeal to in terms of strength. There is a higher father that I appeal to'."[122]

The philosopher Alain de Botton also warns us against excessive optimism. Like Atul Gawande, he thinks a degree of pessimism can actually reduce the distress caused by Fortune's outrageous and unavoidable slings and arrows and reminds us that the churches used to stress the dark side of existence much more than they do now. God knows, there was plenty of darkness before modern medicine, clean water and ways to avoid permanent pregnancy. (The historian author of 'The Age of Agony' asked rhetorically: "Do we realise sufficiently what we have escaped by being alive in the twentieth, not the eighteenth, century?"[123]) De Botton concedes that:

> "We may derive some benefit from the availability of hot baths and computer chips but our lives are no less subject to accident, frustrated ambition, heartbreak, jealousy, anxiety or death than were those of our medieval forebears...[A]t least our ancestors had the advantage of living in a religious era which never made the mistake of promising its population that happiness could ever make a permanent home for itself on this earth."[124] He continues: "If Pascal's pessimism can effectively console us, it may be because we are usually cast into gloom not so much by negativity as by hope. It is hope - with regard to our careers, our love lives, our children, our politicians and our planet - that is primarily to blame for angering and embittering us.... Material improvements since the mid-18th Century have been so remarkable and have so exponentially increased our comfort, safety, wealth and power, as to deal an almost fatal blow to our capacity to remain pessimistic - and therefore, crucially, to our ability to stay sane and content."

John Gray, another philosopher (and, I confess, one of my intellectual heroes) regularly urges his readers and listeners not to assume that 'things can only get better' – the theme tune of New Labour's 1997 election campaign – and also regards faith in the inevitability of 'progress' as a questionable and quasi-religious relic of Enlightenment thinking. "I get the impression with a lot of people – not just the humanists but also the self-professed Christians – that they cling on like grim death to some sort of belief in progress because they really feel that if they give that up, life's not worth living and chaos will break loose. And what I want to say is that this is an unnecessary fear. Epicurus was very cheerful; he was even cheerful when he was dying. You can have a philosophy or view of human life which is positive and cheerful but contains no trace of a belief in human progress."[125] Having seen people lynched during the protests that preceded the 1917 revolution, the Russian-born philosopher, Sir Isaiah Berlin, understood more than many people that history was not an inevitable arc of progress. He proclaimed:

> "As for the meaning of life, I do not believe that it has any: I do not at all ask what it is, for I suspect it has none, and this is a source of great comfort to me — we make of it what we can, and that is all there is about it. Those who seek for

some deep, cosmic, all-embracing, teleologically arguable libretto or god are, believe me, pathetically deluded."[126]

Nevertheless, his *Times* obituary ended:

> "His was an exuberant life crowded with joys – the joy of thought, the joy of music, the joy of good friends. ... The theme that runs throughout his work is his concern with liberty and the dignity of human beings ... Sir Isaiah radiated well-being."

Attitudes like these stand in stark opposition to a powerful and growing current in Western culture that seeks to protect its citizens against the unpleasant facts of life. TV news programmes regularly feature warnings that 'this item contains images that some people may find disturbing' with the implication that they may also be advised to look away or switch to a more anodyne channel. That may be an appropriate strategy for rearing young children, but it seems an extremely questionable one for adolescents and adults. Resilience is a very desirable component of personality and almost by definition, it fortifies its possessors against unpleasant surprises. To become resilient, real or vicarious exposure to the darker side of life is useful and probably essential. The whole concept of 'safe spaces' in which students of a sensitive disposition can insulate themselves from hearing about the daily horrors of violent crime (and its representations in fiction, drama and courses in criminal law) is an example of that unhelpful inability of human kind to bear much reality. Even among serving soldiers – a group who presumably have little sympathy for 'safe spaces' in ordinary life – a study of paratroopers and Royal Marine commandos with high levels of combat exposure in Iraq and ordinary infantry, found that they "were less likely to have multiple physical symptoms or to be fatigued, and [commandos] also had lower levels of general mental health problems and lower scores on the Post-traumatic Checklist" than ordinary troops. "A possible explanation for this difference is that the *high level of preparedness* in [marines] and [paratroops] may lessen the psychological impact of war-zone deployment experiences"[127] [my italics] A recent study of attitudes to ageing found that in a group of elderly Germans, those with "*more negative views* of older adults in general [had] a lower risk of mortality"[128] [italics original]

That the constructively pessimistic view of life advised by writers like de Botton, Gawande and Gray is not only realistic but also protective against psychological disorder is further suggested by the few studies that have examined the concept of 'trauma vaccination'. That analogy is a close one, for just as vaccination with a milder form of an infection enables vaccine recipients to withstand or avoid the full disease, so does deliberate exposure to the *idea* of traumatic events and to images of real and simulated disasters seem to help recipients to deal more effectively with real-life traumas by rehearsing possible responses. So far, clinical studies have been restricted to victims of torture[129] and to civil defence workers.[130] The torture study indicated that political activists who regarded torture as a significant possibility, and were thus to some extent prepared for it, had fewer subsequent problems than those who were tortured even though they had not been involved in politics. All military training involves not merely psychological and logistical preparation for conflict but also the most realistic possible simulation of real conflict short of inflicting real wounds. I want my airline pilot to be factually and emotionally prepared and equipped for every conceivable flying disaster. I do not want the recruitment of surgeons to become difficult because future medical schools feel obliged, in the interests of diversity, to accommodate medical students who cannot cope with blood and other body fluids.

Ehrenreich mostly passes over the prayers that irritated Amy-Claire and that were frequently mentioned on the breast cancer website but life remains uncertain and the god that Amy Claire's fellow-sufferers want her to pray to and to thank for his allegedly helpful therapeutic interventions used to be even more ineffective than he seems to be today. In prosperous, well-doctored societies like ours, even young people get illnesses that ruin their lives or kill them: sometimes both. It is not only those of a religious disposition who find this state of affairs hard to contemplate and harder still to come to terms with.

Personally, I have never regarded mortality as a problem since I was a child and I remember precisely the moment when it both started and stopped causing me distress. It was around the end of the war, so I must have been four years old. The bombs and air-raid sirens that regularly punctuated my earliest recollections had ceased. I had gone to bed but downstairs, my parents had invited some friends to dinner, perhaps to celebrate the approach of peace in Europe. Quite suddenly, the thought came into my head that everyone dies and that I too would one day be dead. I don't know what caused this epiphany. Nobody close to me had died or become seriously ill and I don't think the particularly murderous nature of WW2 had penetrated my awareness. Whatever the reasons, the thought upset me and like any young mammal in distress, I called to my mother for comfort. Within two minutes, and without any training in grief management or the other arts of the not-yet-named counselling professions, she dealt with my fears. It was true, she acknowledged, that we are all going to die but if it were really such a serious concern, she and my father - being nearer to death than I - ought to be much more upset than I was. As for my grandmothers, then nearing three-score-and-ten ... These sensible and practical points made, she returned to the guests and left me wiser and happier. She would surely have endorsed the point made in a philosophical volume that: "Every single person now alive will be dead in the not too distant future. This fact is universally accepted and is not seen as remarkable, still less as an impending catastrophe. There are no crisis meetings of world leaders to consider what to do about it, no outbreaks of mass hysteria, no outpourings of grief, no demands for action ... Not only is that fact not regarded as a catastrophe, it is not even on anybody's list of the major problems facing the world."[131] I don't think my mother had read much about the Victorian scientist Michael Faraday, though she liked Victorian novelists but I am reminded of his famous response to the woman who said to him: "Mr Faraday, I accept the universe". "My god, madam," he is said to have replied, "you'd better!"

If you believe in a benevolent deity, it tends to follow that you believe he is trying to make life pleasant, at least for those who worship him in the right way, otherwise why bother with intercessionary prayer? Over the centuries, many Christians have wrestled with the Problem of Evil. Explaining why the wicked prosper and why pain and horrible diseases exist in a supposedly good and beautiful world ('the best of all possible worlds' as claimed by Leibnitz and satirised by Voltaire in *Candide*)[132] gave rise to a large and historically important chunk of theology called theodicy. If we don't hear much about it these days, perhaps it is because the churches have come up with no new ideas and the old ones are increasingly seen as unconvincing or irrelevant.

Let us look at how ordinary people, and more particularly ordinary patients, deal with the business of dying. Many of them have little in the way of specific as opposed to vague and general religious belief, yet they have to deal with the fact that their lives will soon be over. Firm religious belief can be a comfort to the dying but the nature of the religion's defining and fundamental doctrines is usually unimportant. Being religious, in a general sense, may be helpful but only in a placebo-like, non-specific way. There is no evidence that belief in Christian doctrines, for example, helps more than belief in the doctrines of other faiths, yet those doctrines are the core of inter-religious (and intra-religious) disputes. They are the crucial components that missionaries for Religion

A claim gives their religion specific advantages over Religion B, or over unbelief, just as drug A may be better than drug B, or a placebo. Defenders of religion often assert that church membership protects against many conditions and afflictions in addition to the distress of dying and mortality, ranging from mental illness and reduced life-expectancy to involvement in crime and drug abuse. There are studies that may appear to show this but the important component, which is to say, the active or specifically 'therapeutic' component, turns out not to be membership of any particular faith but membership of certain kinds of group. "Religious affiliates may see themselves as more moral, and priming their religious affiliation did indeed induce greater morality, but this was also true for other social affiliations. Therefore, religion is not fundamental to moral priming, and it is likely to be *the perceived benefits of being in a group* that enhances prosociality."[133] [my italics] That may explain why "The negative association between religion and substance use/abuse is not limited to traditional religious groups". In the 20th century, active membership of a Communist, Nationalist or Fascist party, as well as cults and street-gangs, provided powerful and subjectively positive group solidarity and conformity-encouraging effects, as many memoirs of the period testify. Active members of a church, or an AA group, get some benefit simply from the group support that membership provides, as well as from specific religious activities such as prayer and other rituals. It is one more variety of religious behaviour whose benefits can be parsimoniously explained by non-specific and placebo effects without invoking the specific beliefs of the religion

Sometimes, specific beliefs do provide comfort over and above the non-specific effects or the generalised hope of an afterlife that is not specific to particular religions or even to religion in general. One middle-aged patient was referred to me for a psychiatric opinion by physicians puzzled that he seemed so cheerful despite a creeping paralysis that had left him with bilateral above-knee amputations and a little movement in only one hand. They wondered whether he had brain damage or some other condition that prevented him from appreciating the hopelessness of his predicament but the explanation was much simpler and would have been obvious had they asked him themselves instead of sending him to me to do the asking. He was, he quickly told me, a Christadelphian and thus a member of a dissident sect that had implanted in him the firm belief that his current phase of existence was only a prelude to something very much better, in which his amputated limbs and lost functions would be restored. Unlike mainstream Christian sects, Christadelphians do not believe in the immortality of the soul. Instead, they believe that after a period of non-existence, they will be resurrected in the flesh to share a perfect physical world with the resurrected Christ. The same certainties about future pleasures that enable Islamist suicide bombers to face death with equanimity or enthusiasm can have similar useful effects in the terminally ill but fewer and fewer people in Britain outside the major ethnic minorities now have firm beliefs of that kind. [134]

In any case, a major disadvantage of that sort of belief is that in real life (and real death) not everyone can be certain of resurrection. That was a serious and terrifying concern for the great Dr Samuel Johnson. According to his biographer Boswell:

> "Dr. Johnson surprised [Mr. Henderson] not a little, by acknowledging with a look of horror, that he was much oppressed by the fear of death. The amiable Dr. Adams suggested that God was infinitely good. *Johnson:* 'That he is infinitely good, as far as the perfection of his nature will allow, I certainly believe; but it is necessary for good upon the whole, that individuals should be punished. As to an *individual,* therefore, he is not infinitely good; and as I cannot be *sure* that I have fulfilled the conditions on which salvation is granted, I am afraid I may be one of those who shall be damned' (looking dismally). *Dr. Adams:* 'What do you mean by damned?' *Johnson:* (passionately and loudly) 'Sent to Hell, Sir, and punished everlastingly'."

When Peter Hitchens, Christoper Hitchens's journalist brother and a *Marxisant* unbeliever at the time, found himself in front of Rogier van der Weyden's altarpiece in the Hospices de Beaune, its vivid depiction of the punishments of the wicked made him suddenly feel frightened and uncomfortable and apparently continues to do so.[135] He had "...absolutely no doubt that I was among the damned, if there were any damned". Within a few months, he had rejoined the Church of England, against whose modernised, damnation-lite services, "its bishops, its arid modern prayers and poetry-free, unmemorable modern bibles ... its stripped and carpeted modernised churches, its compulsory handshakes, perky modern hymns or happy-clappy conventicles where everyone is saved", he now profitably fulminates.[136] I share some of his traditionalist criticisms but for aesthetic rather than theological reasons. The large number of people who simply prefer not to think too much about these things, and for whom neither belief nor disbelief have been important, may be troubled by similar Johnsonian (and Hitchensian) doubts in their final days. This sort of theological fence-sitting can cause problems in other areas of life as well. Albert Ellis, the lapsed Freudian who developed Rational-Emotive Behaviour Therapy, an alternative talking-and-listening approach, called them 'ecclesial neuroses'. They can be seen as adverse intellectual effects of religious belief and sometimes, they can be quite serious. "Faith" it has been said "is the fatigue resulting from the attempt to preserve God's integrity instead of one's own."[137] Unfortunately, Marx's famous religion-as-opiate analogy has two facets. Religion can provide relief from existential anxiety but like opiates, it frequently causes addiction and dependence, leading to extremely unpleasant withdrawal symptoms that many victims will do anything to avoid, even if that means committing offences against truth and logic in order to maintain their dysfunctional intellectual habit. I was not surprised when a very recent study reported that the personal characteristics most strongly associated with a belief in Complementary and Alternative medicine are 'belief [in] Life after Death ... Religiousness ... and Optimism'.[138] Significantly, patients can become addicted to pure placebos in ways very similar to the development of tolerance and addiction to opiates, needing larger doses to get the same effects and showing marked withdrawal symptoms when their supply of placebos was interrupted.[139]

Definite unbelievers, on the other hand, don't seem to find the prospect of annihilation as distressing as many believers do. Baron d'Holbach, the discreet Enlightenment atheist, was relaxed about his prospects and about how soon he would be forgotten, as indeed he largely has been:

> "The Corneilles, the Lockes, the Newtons, the Boyles, the Harveys, the Montesquieus, the Sheridans are no more! Regretted by a small number of friends, who have presently [i.e. quickly] consoled themselves by their necessary avocations, their death was indifferent to the greater number of their fellow citizens. Darest thou then flatter thyself, that thy reputation, thy titles, thy riches, thy sumptuous repasts, thy diversified pleasures, will make thy funeral a melancholy event! It will be spoken of by some few for two days, and do not be at all surprised: learn that there have died in former ages, in Babylon, in Sardis, in Carthage, in Athens, in Rome, millions of citizens more illustrious, more powerful, more opulent, more voluptuous, than thou art; of whom, however, no one has taken care to transmit to thee even the names."[140]

In other words: 'get over it'. I think Alain de Botton, Atul Gawande and John Gray would agree.

Phil Zuckerman, a Californian sociologist of religion, spent a study year in Denmark. After his surprise at how small a place religion seemed to have in Danish life compared with anywhere in the US, he started conducting surveys of Danish attitudes to such fundamental questions as dying and The Meaning of Life. One of his informants was Anne, a hospice nurse who, like many Danes, combined an absence of conventional religious belief with membership of the national (Lutheran) church and payment of its annual membership tax. Reluctant to describe herself as an atheist, she said that she tried to live "in a Christian way" by which she meant "not to steal, be kind to all people and so on". She was not so unbelieving that she dismissed the idea of reincarnation or of the existence of a soul and had experienced some strange feelings and sensations at the moment when patients died. Most of her hospice patients were not religious and died without requesting any religious attention. The few who took their Christianity seriously were mainly very old and they seemed to have Dr Johnson's problem. "It's very difficult for them to die. They are afraid of dying. They are afraid that God doesn't take them to heaven and they are thinking of their life and have they done something wrong". Asked whether people without religion had similar problems, she replied, "No, it's the Christians who have problems". Larger surveys tend to support her anecdotal report that atheists generally cope well with death, though it is likely that "firmness and consistency of beliefs and practices, rather than religiousness per se, are buffers against death anxiety in old age".[141] The same study found that "Individuals who were moderately religious feared death more than individuals who scored high or low on religiousness", as did a large recent meta-analysis.[142] This is similar to an observation by one of my gynaecology teachers, talking about contraception and pre-marital sex in the 1960s. "It's not 'good' girls who get pregnant, because they don't have sex and it's not 'bad' girls, because they take precautions. It's the *demi-vierges* [the semi-virgins] who get pregnant because they tell themselves they're not going to have sex and then when they do, they aren't prepared for it, because being prepared would mean admitting the possibility that they could be 'bad'." Both happily sceptical unbelievers and happily convinced believers like my Christadelphian patient are more relaxed about death than the many theological *demi-vierges* who don't take psychological precautions because that means having to think about the possibility of dying. In the same way, believers who are certain that the atheists are wrong may be less worried than those who have sneaking fears that the atheists may be right. The 17th century theologian Jacques Bernard was "afraid that [atheist writings] would disclose thoughts to me that would throw me into a fear from which I would not be able to return" and his contemporary André d'Abillon felt that for such sceptics, "there is no punishment violent enough for so dark a crime'.[143] However, to be a happy believer when nearing death, you may also have to be convinced that you have lived a life free of sins or that if you haven't, God will nevertheless forgive you. That may not be easy. Baron d'Holbach noted the paradox that while "the goodness of God cheers the wicked, his rigour disturbs the honest man." Happy unbelievers are spared that problem.

Zuckerman did manage to find some religious Danes (including a very laid-back pastor) but Denmark, followed closely by Sweden, has the world's highest proportion of unbelievers in any kind of personal god – probably around 75%. Barely 20% thought that God was fairly or very important in their life. The percentage who regarded the bible as the literal word of God was in single figures. Despite this widespread rejection of religion, many Danes and Swedes pay their church tax, as Anne did but this is usually because of residual Nordic tribal loyalties. It is "what Danes do" and for the same essentially tribal, unreligious and aesthetic reasons, many Danes are confirmed and get married in church and have their children baptised there. They may get buried there too but apart from these occasions, they never take part in church services. Zuckerman could hardly avoid noticing that Denmark and Sweden (and Norway) are also among the least violent, corrupt and unequal societies on the planet and have excellent universal health systems. They have more women in public life than most countries and give proportionately more aid to poor countries. Danes regularly come top in international lists of happiness and satisfaction with life. When Danes were asked what were the most important qualities to foster in their children, "87% chose "tolerance/respect", 80% chose "independence", 72% "good manners", 56% "to think of others" and 37% "imagination". Only 8% chose "Christian faith".' It is in this context that we should not be surprised at the results of a recent survey that studied altruism and sharing behaviour in children from religious (Muslim and Christian) or non-religious families. The latter scored more highly. "[R]eligiousness was inversely predictive of children's altruism and positively correlated with their punitive tendencies. Together these results reveal the similarity across countries in how religion negatively influences children's altruism, challenging the view that religiosity facilitates prosocial behavior'.[144]

What 'Christianity' means to most Danes has nothing to do with the central doctrines of the church – Christ's crucifixion and atonement for our sins, the Eucharist, resurrection and eternal life. It means the 'golden rule' – doing unto others as you would have them do unto you (though George Bernard Shaw joked that we shouldn't, because "other people's tastes might be different"). The golden rule was worked out and written down long before Jesus is supposed to have mentioned it and most commentators feel that no revelations, or great insights into human nature, were needed to bring that about.

Yet the leaders of most religions regularly assert or imply that people without a religion can have no purpose in life and no moral compass. Lord Sacks, the former Chief Rabbi and one of our unelected legislators until his death, claimed the non-religious view means that: "There is nothing whatsoever that distinguishes us qualitatively from the animal kingdom or any other life form. All ideals are illusions, all hopes are destined to be destroyed and life has no meaning whatsoever."[145] Like Sir Isaiah Berlin, most of the Danes Zuckerman interviewed denied that there was any religious, cosmic, overall purpose or meaning in life but they seemed well equipped with both purposes and morals. Life, whatever existential questions it threw up, was something they got on with. Their family, work and leisure were important. They tried to enjoy life and to help others enjoy it (especially their families and friends) and most of them tried to make the world a better place in small or sometimes more ambitious ways.

Does that make them worse people than Lord Sacks? They regarded their loss of religion as simply a matter of growing up. "I heard – time after time ... that their belief in God simply withered with age, undramatically and without much to do. ... The notion that religious belief is somehow childish, that faith in God is just something that one dabbles with in childhood but eventually grows out of as one becomes a mature adult, would strike most Americans as offensive. But for millions of Scandinavians, that's just the way it is".

That is consistent with formal studies in the psychology of religion. A particularly revealing one compared 'Amazing Apostates' with 'Amazing Believers'. Both groups were 'amazing' because they had either been brought up in religious families but had become unbelievers, or vice versa. Since the subjects were university students, the change, in both groups, had mostly taken place during their teens but the time-scale and the reasons were very different. Amazing Apostates began to question religion as they began to question many other things around or before the age of puberty. It usually took them several years before their questioning reached the stage of rejection. "Many ... reported initial guilt and fear about dropping their religious beliefs ... [Their] explanations typically revolved around their need to ask questions and get answers, their intellectual curiosity and their unwillingness to accept responses that they felt did not really answer their questions. Most ... had spent considerable time and effort weighing different arguments for and against religious beliefs ... [they] were 'amazing' in [their rejection of childhood/socializing influences] through an intellectual search for truth in their own lives".

In telling contrast, Amazing Believers were likely to have 'found religion' in an attempt to deal with crises in their lives. Emotional issues such as fear, loneliness and depression seemed to drive their amazing conversion (as they may drive placebo responses to treatment for frightening illnesses). For example, some were attempting to escape from dependence on drugs, alcohol or sex; other were grappling with serious illness or tragedy in their lives. One woman who became an Amazing Believer had had four close relatives and friends die tragically in one year.[146] Another difference was that Amazing Apostates "... held very tolerant, non-authoritarian attitudes towards others, in contrast to their highly religious [Amazing Believers] counterparts". Zuckerman's finding that the largely non-religious Danes typically valued independence and tolerance begins to look like a causal relationship.

The major textbook of the psychology of religion that is the source of these quotations is full of interesting and sometimes unexpected research findings. "The data are clear: Women consistently demonstrate a greater affinity for religion than men."[p 153] Using a 'secret survey' technique, a researcher was surprised to find that "about one third of his participants who were high in right-wing authoritarianism admitted that they had *secret* doubts about God's existence - doubts that they had *never* shared with anyone else."[p 134] "Apparently cheating is quite widespread among high-school and college students and it does not seem to make much difference whether or not students are religious....[Earlier research] found essentially no relationship between religion and honesty or cheating. In fact, there was even some tendency for children who attended Sunday school to be less cooperative and helpful". [p 419-20] "In view of the clear teachings of most faiths on such issues, we are left to ponder why religion does not have a significant impact in reducing cheating *behaviour*". [p 422] 'Batson et al (1973) concluded that "this evidence strongly suggests that the more religious show no more active concern for others than do the less religious. The more religious only present themselves as more concerned". [p 125] All italics are original. However, when you get involved in arguments with believers, bear in mind that "Twin studies suggest that about half the variation in scores on religious measures was broadly genetic."[p 54] And while Danes may not get much comfort from the idea of God, I imagine that most of them are comforted by placebo effects.

Furthermore, even Danes are probably not immune to what three American psychologists, who appear to be the authorities on a concept known as 'Terror Management Theory' call 'The worm at the core'[147] – a phrase they took from their great American psychological predecessor William James's 'Varieties of Religious Experience'. That 'worm' is death; our attitudes to it, our fear and denial of it and our reluctance to engage with it and accept it. They share my view of the importance of death and disease in the development of religion in our ancestors, who "ingeniously conspired to 'just say no' to reality by creating a supernatural universe that *afforded a sense of control over life and death,* enabling them to bound over the 'yawning chasm' and cross the cognitive Rubicon that triggered humankind's evolutionary explosion". (my italics) Whether or not you accept the broader implications of their research, the most impressive thing about it is the way it shows beyond reasonable doubt that the observable behaviour of ordinary people is profoundly and predictably affected by reminders of death of which they are not consciously aware. As well as judges who increased the fine almost tenfold in a judicial sentencing simulation after subliminal exposure to intimations of mortality, Christians apparently become "more intent on persuading atheists to embrace Jesus" after similar reminders. However, the same reminders also "make evolutionists more determined to persuade creationists to embrace Darwin". The authors' explanation is that persuading someone to accept your beliefs makes us "more confident of their validity" and consequently less worried about our own death. Whatever the explanation, it seems likely that subconscious anxieties about death are common and lurk in the background of many medical consultations, even for minor illnesses.

To maintain, as I do in Chapter 18, that psychoanalysis and its allied cults do not provide insights into the 'subconscious' that are both true and therapeutically useful is not the same as saying that the subconscious does not exist and the Terror Management experiments confirm that it does. Prof Kaptchuk's team also showed that subconscious cues could increase or decrease pain perception,[148] which adds to the evidence that subconscious and symbolic factors strongly influence placebo responses. However, that is a long way from developing techniques to make people less worried about death, or from showing that it would be a good thing if we could. By the time most people get to the age when they have good reason to worry about their health, their personalities are well-established and difficult to change except in rather marginal ways. One of the Terror Management researchers, Tom Pyszczynski, told me that there was no research that assesses the effect of death reminders on placebo effects but that some as yet unpublished studies "suggest that viewing death with an attitude of acceptance or curiosity might reduce defensive reactions to it". Perhaps we can add that to the list of things that distinguish doctors from the majority of citizens. For example, we *attempt* suicide very much less often than the general public but our rate of *completed* suicide is not very different. While there are probably at least twenty attempts in the general population for every completed suicide, there are relatively few unsuccessful attempts among doctors.[149] We tend to do it properly or not at all. It may be significant that US doctors, who are about as likely as the general US population to believe in God, are less likely to believe in an afterlife and much more likely to "make sense of the situation and decide what to do without relying on God".[150]

Like many modern philosophers and scientists, including John Gray, Sir Isaiah Berlin and Richard Dawkins, I am more at ease than Charles Darwin was with the powerful and growing evidence that the existence of *homo sapiens* is essentially a random event in a random universe. If they think about it at all, people who are troubled or terrified by that idea generally either come to terms with it or seek solace in a religion that gives the hope of a creator-god and an afterlife, if those evidence-lite hypotheses have not already been irremovably implanted in childhood. In any case, by the time people start to think about such things, staying alive has usually become an extremely powerful and unthinking habit, powerfully reinforced by networks of relationships and responsibilities. Nevertheless, the randomness does make a few people feel more than transiently suicidal. I have interviewed many failed suicides and in my clinical experience, this tiny and atypical group were almost invariably male, usually in their late teens or early twenties and not infrequently formal or informal students of philosophy; or aspiring writers. Despite Albert Camus' most famous one-liner ("There is but one truly serious philosophical problem, and that is suicide.") remarkably few of these questioners get as far as ending their lives. About 1% of UK deaths are due to suicide. World-wide, the proportion attributable to taking Monsieur Camus too seriously is vanishingly small.[151]

'Acceptance or curiosity' are among the words I would use to describe my own attitude to death, for which I probably have to thank both my mother and my medical education. Although hospital doctors in particular seem to find it difficult to avoid resuscitating moribund patients with a poor prognosis, many doctors would not want such procedures if they themselves were in that position.[152] Most British potential patients don't want them either but those of non-European ethnicity, who tend to be more religious, are much more likely to say they would want to be resuscitated even if they were in the terminal stages of dementia.[153] So do atypically religious Dutch Protestant patients.[154]

Chapter 11
Remind me: why won't God help amputees?
The attraction of prayers for recovery – and the reality

20% of people admit to regular prayer of a broadly intercessional kind – half of them daily. Many report feeling better and calmer and believe it makes a difference to what actually happens.
BBC news item for Sunday 12th Nov 2007 - Remembrance Sunday for the dead of two world wars
Religion. Church of England (if you really must). This is a quiet and decent superstition, as they go, offering a wide choice in decoration and no poisonous enthusiasms.
Simon Raven. Letter to my Son. The Spectator, 10 Mar 1967

One Sunday morning soon after qualifying, I was attending to a patient in, shall we say, Ward 5 when the hospital's Anglican chaplain arrived for his regular Sunday visit. The curtains were already drawn around my patient's bed and therefore the chaplain and I could not see each other but I could hardly avoid overhearing him. What he said seemed pretty standard Anglican stuff and he presumably said much the same in all the other wards he visited. It was only his final supplication that struck me as rather farcical, though no doubt comforting to the less philosophically sophisticated patients. "And give thy blessing, O Lord, especially," he intoned, "to the patients in Ward 5". John Betjeman satirized this kind of special pleading perfectly in his wartime poem 'In Westminster Abbey' with the punch-line:

'Lord, put beneath Thy special care
One eighty-nine Cadogan Square'.[155]

More thoughtful clerics are evidently aware of a principle known to all health economists; namely, that with finite budgets, giving special treatment and resources to one group of patients inevitably means taking resources away from another group. The following reported conversation took place between a priest and a parishioner sheltering in the basement of an East End vicarage during the London blitz:

"I asked a woman whether she prayed when she heard a bomb falling. 'Yes', she answered; 'I pray: Oh God! Don't let it fall here'. 'But', I said, 'it's a bit rough on the other people, if your prayer is granted, and the thing drops, not on you, but on them'. 'I can't help that', she replied. 'They must say their prayers and push it off further'."[156]

The hospital chaplain was only asking his tribal Anglican God to help in a general sort of way but many sick or unhappy people and many clerics are much more specific in their requests for divine intercession. A few years ago, while walking in the centre of Melbourne, I wandered into St Paul's Anglican cathedral and before leaving, I picked up a leaflet entitled 'Healing Prayer: what's it all about?'. It didn't go into much detail, suggesting that people who wanted more information should telephone the leader of the 'Healing Ministry Team' but it did make a few very specific claims. 'Does God always answer? He does!' After cautioning that God might first require supplicants to do a little preparatory work, such as 'to change their lifestyle or repent [or] forgive someone who's hurt them' it continues: 'But in the time of prayer, in some way God will begin something wonderful in your life. There is nothing you cannot ask God to help with. If you trust him and open the door to him, he *can* act'. (emphasis original.) I didn't get the impression that St Paul's was unusually gung-ho about divine healing. It seemed pretty mainstream and relaxed in the Anglo-Anglican (as opposed to Afro-Anglican) fashion and if it espoused any of Simon Raven's 'poisonous enthusiasms', they were not on view that day.[157] The Jesuit priest Jean Grou was more confident that God not only '*can*' but definitely will act. "If there is one single thing on which our Lord insisted frequently and with the utmost force and lucidity, it is the efficacy of prayer. In one place he said: *All things whatsoever ye shall ask in prayer, believing, ye shall receive.*"[158] (italics original) Had I wandered into Melbourne's Roman Catholic cathedral instead, I would have encountered a culture in which intercessionary prayer is a much more prominent activity and regularly reinforced by the creation of new saints whose canonisation or even preliminary beatification requires them to have performed miracles, nearly always of a therapeutic nature.

There are, in reality, many things that God either can't do, or can do but won't do, however fervently and frequently people pray to him, however many holy relics they touch and however much incense priests burn on their behalf. (Or, until the mid-19th century, however many *castrati*, genitally mutilated before puberty, were recruited into the Vatican choir, the better to sing the praises of the Catholic God.) George Bernard Shaw was perhaps the most famous but not the first visitor to observe that although discarded crutches and splints were easy to find at Lourdes and other places of therapeutic pilgrimage, there was a telling absence of discarded artificial limbs and glass eyes. One well-travelled commentator wrote: "I have visited Lourdes in France and Fatima in Portugal, healing shrines of the Christian Virgin Mary. I have also visited Epidaurus in Greece and Pergamum in Turkey, healing shrines of the pagan god Asklepios. The miraculous healings recorded in both places were remarkably the same. There are, for example, many crutches hanging in the grotto of Lourdes, mute witness to those who arrived lame and left whole. There are, however, no prosthetic limbs among them..."[159] For some reason, no deity – old or new – has ever convincingly restored a limb or an eye that has been removed by surgery or injury, particularly in the last century or so when x-ray or photographic records could have supported any such claim. It really does seem as if God excludes amputees from miraculous healing. (There is an informative website devoted to the phenomenon.[160])

This is, on the face of it, puzzling and disappointing. Several animal species - starfish, stone-crabs and lizards, for example - are able to regrow limbs or tails that have been lost to predators or accidents. Indeed, the tasty stone crab obligingly and consistently grows a new and bigger claw if fishermen harvest one and then return the crab to the ocean. Furthermore, traditional depictions of the two major patron saints of healing – Saints Cosmas and Damian – show them grafting a leg onto a man who has had a below-knee amputation. We can be sure that it was not the man's own leg that was being sewn back on, remarkable though that would have been for surgery in the pre-aseptic and pre-antibiotic age, because although the patient is white, the grafted leg is not. (In some paintings, its original owner is depicted in the background.) A few sceptics have even suggested a simple and persuasive clinical trial, in which large numbers of Christians, Moslems, Hindus etc, would agree to pray on a particular day for missing limbs to be restored to a group of well-documented amputees. Even a single independently verified re-grown arm or leg would be a sensational event. That trial has yet to be organized but following the canonization of Mother Teresa of Calcutta in 2016, an enthusiastic Catholic academic called Benjamin Wiker publicly urged millions of the faithful to pray not only for the recovery and 'complete healing' of the unbelieving physicist Stephen Hawking from muscular dystrophy but also for his conversion to Catholicism. Wiker, a professor of political science at a Catholic university in the USA, called for mass prayers "during [Mother Teresa's] canonization day, and eight days thereafter".[161] Hawking remained unhealed and unconverted until his death in 2018.

Just how generally unconvincing are the claims of medical miracles wrought by candidates for sainthood, recorded since the 13th century and kept in the Vatican, emerges from a study by Prof Jacalyn Duffin, who is both a haematologist and a historian of medicine.[162] In the former capacity, she was asked in the 1980s to look at a series of bone marrow slides without, at first, being told why – in other words, 'blind' to the clinical background. She "found this to be a case of severe acute leukaemia with a remission, a relapse, and another remission" and assumed that the patient was dead and that she was being asked for a medico-legal report. It turned out that the patient was very much alive; and that despite having had appropriate anti-leukaemic medication, she had attributed her recovery not to the medication but to intercession by Marie-Marguerite d'Youville, a Montreal woman who had died two hundred years earlier. As a historian, Prof. Duffin was naturally delighted to learn that her microscopic skills would provide evidence for the process of canonization of d'Youville as the first Canadian-born saint. Eventually, she was invited to the Vatican, met the Pope (John Paul II) and was granted access to relevant parts of the Vatican Secret Archive. Over three subsequent visits, she tried to answer some obvious questions. Such as: "What diseases were cured? How many miracles, like 'mine', entailed cutting-edge science and the testimony of sceptical, even atheist, physicians like me?"

One of her main interests was how these cases changed over the centuries[163] and that is certainly an interesting aspect of miracle cures, naturally reflecting changes in both medical and popular perceptions of disease. The rules of the game are, apparently, that it's God, rather than the putative, wannabe saint, who works the miracles. The saint merely intercedes with God on behalf of those who request saintly assistance. Such confidence in the precise mechanism of healing is not always found even in modern medicine. Direct reports from either the treating physician or other medical witnesses of the time were rarer before the 17th century but in 1949, Pope Pius XII set up the *Consulta Medica* to provide expert advice, though it mainly just formalised arrangements that had existed since the 19th century. Membership is prestigious and "restricted to distinguished physicians, mostly male academics from Rome, who are practising Catholics. They are paid honoraria for their contributions". In subsequent email correspondence, Prof. Duffin chided me gently for suggesting that the requirement that they be practising Catholics (and presumably, believing ones too, as far as that could be judged) might adversely affect their objectivity. Although an atheist herself, she also claimed that my preference for non-supernatural, scientific explanations was itself "a parallel belief system" but that is a common misunderstanding and one more often heard from theists on the defensive than from a self-described atheist. The scientific method – the basis of scientific explanations - is not a belief system. It is just a well-tried and constantly refined method for evaluating truth claims, especially conflicting truth claims. To the extent that 'science' pronounces for or against certain claims (or answers – as religions rarely do - 'don't know') it is using concepts of evidence that should apply equally to all truth claims; religious, biochemical, anatomical, geological or any other kind. Quite apart from the question of which god they have in mind, religious apologists cannot simply assert with justified confidence that 'God exists' or 'God did it' without having to answer the very simple question: 'How do you know that?' (or alternatively, 'what would disprove your claim?') and accepting, as the null hypothesis requires, that it is their job to prove the claim rather than for doubters to disprove it. Given that miracles, medical or otherwise are, by definition, 'extraordinary', they should also observe the convention that 'extraordinary claims require extraordinary evidence'. Otherwise, anything goes.

Eventually, Prof. Duffin had access to some 1400 miracles from several hundred saints since 1600 for study. At least two miracles have to be attested but Pope John-Paul II reduced the role and power of the Devil's Advocate, whose traditional job is to question the evidence, and seems to have preferred saintly quantity to saintly quality. Within less than two decades after becoming pope, he had presided over the canonisation or beatification of nearly 1500 people. This massive expansion of the Vatican's saint-factory has created more saints than the entire total "since Pope Urban VIII started the formal process in the 1620s."[164] Prof. Duffin initially concentrated on the final miracle, on the basis that "the miracle immediately preceding the decision to canonize must have been somewhat convincing – at least, it could not have been unconvincing". That covered over a third of all the miracles in the files. Interestingly, a miracle would not be pronounced if a sick person had rejected medical advice, even at a time when it was very unlikely to have been specifically useful, and had sought only divine intervention. Clearly, the Vatican shared the general and mistaken belief in the effectiveness of doctors.

Some 4% were not strictly medical and half of this subgroup involved the 'miraculous' preservation of the saint's corpse, though most of these saints were credited with ordinary healing miracles as well. As Prof. Duffin notes, bodily preservation without formal mummification "is now considered to occur within the realm of natural possibility and is insufficient evidence for a canonization miracle". As one might expect, the earlier the miracle, the more likely it was that the condition involved was something obvious to the naked eye and to layman and physician alike, if indeed a physician was on hand. That meant mainly skin diseases, fevers, blindness, convulsions, paralysis and lameness, since the internal organs were not usually visible in life and their functions (and disorders of function) hardly began to be understood until well into the 19th century. Spontaneous recovery from all these conditions can and does occur, depending on the underlying cause. As for tumours, it would have been almost impossible to distinguish between the spontaneous rupture and disappearance of an alarming but not life-threatening cyst inside the abdomen and the disappearance of a solid abdominal mass whose malignant or non-malignant nature could not be known. Spontaneous recovery is especially likely when the paralysis, convulsion or blindness is due to hysteria (a.k.a. psychogenic, conversion or somatoform disorder) a condition that can still cause diagnostic confusion and was much commoner in less sophisticated societies. It gets a detailed discussion in Chapter 15.

Cancer had been recognised for millennia but not everything that looks cancerous is malignant, in the sense of spreading or 'metastasising' to distant organs or invading them directly. Spontaneous remission or disappearance of cancer is rare but well documented and happens to the prayerful and the unprayerful alike. Slow-growing malignancies are not uncommon in late life, including many prostate cancers and some breast cancers. As we say in the trade, you usually die *with* them, not *from* them. With modern diagnostic techniques like those Prof. Duffin used to confirm the leukaemia, we can at least be fairly confident about a specific diagnosis of cancer, yet in some conditions, it can be difficult to distinguish malignant cells from non-malignant ones of similar appearance, even with the benefit of hindsight. A paper tellingly entitled "'Patients with terminal cancer' who have neither terminal illness nor cancer" described a patient whose lung biopsy was diagnosed microscopically by two independent pathologists as showing a particularly malignant cancer, possibly originating in a primary cancer of the hip. When after seven months he was not dying as expected, he was reassessed. The hip turned out to be arthritic rather than cancerous and was successfully replaced but when a third pathologist reviewed the original biopsy slides, he too thought the cells looked malignant.[165] The authors described three further cases of essentially spontaneous (and potentially 'miraculous') recovery from what looked like terminal cancer but wasn't. Ironically, soon after her unexpected recovery, one of the patients developed a real cancer that killed her within a couple of years.

Here are a few more case reports of 'miraculous' cures without any obvious divine intervention. In 2007, Dutch doctors reported two cases of spontaneous remission of a type of leukaemia in which remissions are usually very rare and short-lived.[166] In both cases, the patients had experienced the sort of severe chest infection that at one time would often have been fatal by itself. They speculate that infections might trigger an immune response that may, very occasionally, abort leukaemia and other cancers. Two similar cases involved remissions of leukaemia for 34 and 17 months following severe pneumonia.[167,168] Another patient with a rare leukaemia had been in remission for 12 years without treatment, after getting infected with hepatitis from one of the many blood transfusions he received.[169] In a pre-antibiotic age, the co-existence of cancer with a severe infection would have been commoner.

If we look at malignant tumours rather than malignant blood disorders, similar unexpected disappearances are not difficult to find. A 1997 review[170] found over 60 reports since 1964 of the spontaneous disappearance of secondary, metastatic tumours from kidney cancer, including metastatic tumours in bone, liver, lung and brain. A 68-year-old woman had a breast lump that grew from 1cm to 2.5cms in diameter in a few months and was shown to be malignant at biopsy. Surgery had to be delayed for a month because she had an accident but by the time the surgeons operated, the tumour had disappeared and although tissue from the affected area was removed for microscopic examination, no cancer cells were seen in it. "After 78 months of follow-up there was no evidence of relapse."[171] If 60-odd reports over 50 years seems relatively few compared with the number of alleged miracle cures, bear in mind that most doctors don't report cases like this, though they may discuss them at medical meetings and dinner-parties. Writing and submitting papers to medical journals involves much time and effort. Rejection can be terminally discouraging and the major journals rarely accept single case-reports. Young and ambitious junior doctors know this and may regard research papers as more useful for their CVs. Senior doctors do not need to publish in order to further their careers and many are glad that this is so. As the researchers for a Channel 4 TV series pointed out, while almost all cancers occasionally disappear spontaneously, over half the reported cases involve only four types: neuroblastoma (a brain tumour usually found in children) malignant melanoma, choriocarcinoma (a tumour of the placenta) and carcinoma of the kidney.[172]

In other words, even when a diagnosis of cancer has been made with modern diagnostic techniques – the same techniques, presumably, relied on by the Vatican's *Consulta Medica* – malignant tumours do sometimes vanish unexpectedly, often inexplicably and without invoking supernatural means. In a culture where recourse to saints, holy relics and prayer is normal and frequent, it is inevitable that the disappearance of a tumour will sometimes coincide with the performance of a religious ritual, though Pope John-Paul II really did claim, with a level of confidence worthy of President George W. Bush, that "in the designs of Providence, there are no mere coincidences".[173] Coincidences of this kind are much more likely in old accounts where the real nature of the disease in question is not clear to modern physicians. It could have been a disorder that is not generally fatal or progressive, especially when it has a tendency to spontaneous remissions. This must often have been the case until the end of the 19th century and claims of efficacy for saintly intervention were as misleading and mistaken as claims for the effectiveness of most conventional medical treatments of the time. Yet some of the many people who achieved sainthood under Pope John Paul II did so on the basis of these old alleged miracles as well as more recent ones.

It is obviously difficult or impossible to be confident of the real diagnosis in many of the older accounts seen by Prof. Duffin in the archives but not in all. Child-bed fever, due to bacterial infection of the uterus within a few days after childbirth, is not very likely to have been mistaken for a non-infectious condition, or an infection in a very different part of the body. The mortality was high but far from 100% and bacterial infections are notoriously unpredictable. During the Gallipoli campaign of WW1, the poet Rupert Brooke died from infection following a minor insect bite before getting anywhere near the front line. In contrast, Charles XII of Sweden was wounded by a musket ball that passed through his mud-covered boot and shattered several bones in his foot. The subsequent infection was so serious that he was in a coma for a while but he recovered.[174] Prof. Duffin accepts that recent 'miraculous' cures of properly diagnosed neurological conditions such as "epilepsy, multiple sclerosis and myasthenia gravis" could simply reflect the well-recognised occurrence of spontaneous remission in these diseases. "If a cure follows an invocation, sceptics will call it 'coincidence'…they will also expect a relapse." She adds that "Repeated follow-up examinations are usually provided in answer to this concern." However, even in a disease like epilepsy where further attacks are to be expected, lack of relapse without treatment does not prove a miracle, as the following case history shows.

In 1970 while in Australia, I was asked to see a man charged with a double firearm homicide, for which at that time he could have been hanged. The details of the crime are not relevant and are available in published reports[175] but shortly before the offence and for three months afterwards, his behaviour was extremely abnormal. Neither medication nor ECT were helpful, though he recovered by the time of the trial. In what turned out to be the first reported use in a murder trial of the brain x-ray technique that was used before modern scanning techniques appeared a few years later, I was able to show that he had easily visible brain damage in one temporal lobe, probably due to a head injury a few years earlier. There was a pre-homicide history of two brief episodes of confusion. He also had several abnormal electroencephalogram (EEG) recordings after the homicide consistent with a diagnosis of temporal lobe epilepsy (TLE) and there was no adequate motive for the murder. TLE is sometimes associated with psychosis, as in this case, as well as brief seizures; and also with religious fervour and delusions, discussed in Chapter 21. After a verdict of 'not guilty by reason of insanity', he was detained in a secure hospital for five years, during which time he had no medication and no more TLE attacks or psychosis. After his release, I remained in touch with him for another seven TLE-free years; and that is just the experience of one physician who never specialised in epilepsy. Even a brief search of PubMed shows that it is not unique.[176] If the patient's Catholic family had invoked a saint during the period of his profound disturbance, his subsequent spontaneous emergence from that state, the acquittal and his apparently permanent 'cure' could very easily have been judged miraculous.

Unlike alleged miracles, which can only be studied retrospectively, intercessional prayer can be, and has been, subjected to prospective Randomised Controlled Trials. They are easy enough in principle. As with any other medical, surgical or psychological intervention, a sufficient number of patients suffering from a defined condition are randomised to 'treatment' or 'no treatment', which in this context means being prayed for or not being prayed for. Ideally, perhaps, the patients should not know that they were the subjects of an experiment, for then they would have all been equally unaffected by anticipatory concerns that might have had positive or negative effects. These days, patients have to be told and given the opportunity to opt out, though in practice very few refuse. It might be expected that patients who knew or thought that they were being prayed for might have felt more improvement, if only somewhat, than those who weren't sure which group they were in. In the event, one of the better-designed RCTs[177], published in a very reputable journal (and discussed by Richard Dawkins in *The God Delusion*) found that if patients having cardiac by-pass surgery definitely knew that people were praying for them, they had rather more adverse events than those who weren't sure. That may have been because they reasoned that if they were being prayed for, they must really be in a bad way, rather as I suggested earlier might happen to some patients surrounded with lots of bleeping and flashing medical hardware. As with trials of CAM and with clinical trials in general, the more rigorous the design and methodology of the study, the less likely are positive results to be found. Prayer is not exempt from either the Law of Unintended Consequences or the principle that if an intervention can do good, it can also do harm. A different example of its harmful potential may have occurred during the 'Spanish Flu' epidemic of 1918-19. "In Zamora in north-west Spain the bishop ordered a novena – the community was to gather for nine consecutive evenings to pray to St Rocco, patron saint of pestilence, and to kiss his relics." Unfortunately, the gatherings may have facilitated the spread of infection, since it was noted that "Zamoranos seemed to be dying in higher numbers than the residents of other provincial capitals".[178]

Prayer is not restricted to the faithful. People who describe themselves as non-religious by conventional standards also pray after their fashion but they don't seem to pray for any specific benefits. A US survey found that for some of them, "… 'prayer' is primarily a convenient lexical category that overlaps with 'meditation,' 'contemplation,' 'reflection,' and the like. Any spiritual meaning seems thin, submerged in an indistinct mix of reflective practices tied more plainly to personal well-being than to anything much beyond that."[179] Given the evidence from animal studies that differences in handling and other non-specific factors can positively or negatively affect recovery rates from some cancers, we should consider the possibility that the non-specific effects of *any* morale-boosting activity might improve recovery rates in some conditions but morale can be boosted, non-specifically, by both religious and non-religious actions and attitudes.

The only trial that claimed a very significant positive effect of prayer[180] (double the success rate for in-vitro fertilisation) was discredited because:

"Dr. Lobo, identified by the *New York Times* and ABC News as the report's lead author, now claims to have not been involved with the study until after its completion and to have provided only 'editorial assistance'. [His name was subsequently removed from the citation in Pubmed.] Both he and Dr. Cha have refused to respond to phone calls or letters about the study. The remaining author, Daniel Wirth, has no medical degree but has published many studies claiming to support the existence of paranormal phenomena. Many of these studies originated from an entity called, 'Healing Sciences Research International', an organization that he supposedly headed. This entity's only known address was apparently a Post Office box in Orinda, California. Wirth holds an MS degree in the dubious field of 'parapsychology' and also has a law degree.

In April 2004, Wirth and an accomplice (Joseph Horvath) pleaded guilty to conspiracy to commit mail and bank fraud and agreed to forfeit assets of more than $1 million acquired through their schemes. Documents in the case indicate that the pair used assumed names, obtained bogus identifying documents, and obtained employment with a large financial institution from which Horvath improperly paid [monies] to Wirth for alleged services. Wirth's long pattern of dishonest behavior raises several questions about whether the studies in which he was involved actually took place and, if so, whether the results were reported honestly.[181]"

In any case, the Vatican is very strongly opposed to in-vitro fertilisation and therefore the nature of the prayers in this study, if they actually occurred, might have been a very important variable. The patients lived in South Korea, where about a third of the inhabitants are Buddhist, another third Christian and the rest either unbelievers or vaguely shamanistic. Given the Vatican's position on fertility treatment, Catholic prayers might have significantly *reduced* the chances of success.

In the case of prayer studies initiated by believers seeking confirmation rather than sceptics invoking the null hypothesis, there is, as one sceptical commentator notes:

"[An] ...incredible irony of ... 'experiments' involving intercessory prayer. Every one of them has been seeking evidence of a most trivial kind, that could even be mistaken for ... a statistical artefact, from an alleged Power of the most unimaginable magnitude. Power which presumably was the source of the astounding creation of hundreds of billions of galaxies, which are composed of hundreds of trillions of stars, dotted with singularities and 'black holes' possessing immense gravity and crushing annihilatory densities; all of which are dancing with exquisite accuracy in spectacular elliptical orbits over a time- and distance-span of fourteen billion light years ... Meanwhile, they seek evidence of this breathtaking immensity by searching for a measurable difference between the arterial blood flow of a few cardiovascular patients who were prayed for and a few other unfortunates who were not ... a difference in blood pressure between one group of hypertensives who were prayed for and another who were not. It is as if one were asking a composer with a quadrillion times the musical capacity and comprehension of a Ludwig van Beethoven to demonstrate his musicianship by writing out the notes to 'Three Blind Mice'. How petty and insulting to whatever deity these investigators claim to be investigating, when the most they can ask of that which has created biological systems from algae to *sequoia giganticus* and amoebas to human brains [is] 'Let me see if you can fertilize this ovum in a Petri dish with one of your hands tied behind your back'."[182]

This is a field in which, as with CAM, poor experimental design, prejudice (in both directions) and outright fraud are especially high risks. The most recent conclusion of the prestigious Cochrane Collaboration, which analyses results from clinical trials graded according to their quality, transparency and independence, is that: "These findings are equivocal and, although some of the results of individual studies suggest a positive effect of intercessory prayer, the majority do not and the evidence does not support a recommendation either in favour or against the use of intercessory prayer."[183]

Another important similarity between CAM and intercessionary prayer involves the matter of fake medicines, on the one hand, and fake relics on the other. In the case of conventional licensed medicines, quality control of random samples is a crucial and routine aspect of production. Whole batches of a particular medicine are occasionally withdrawn when they are found to be sub-standard because patients' lives may depend on receiving the correct dosage. In medicines that are essentially placebos, dosage is usually irrelevant unless one or more of the components is toxic and, in any case, how can the prescriber become suspicious of a particular batch when neither the genuine herbal article nor an inferior fake could have any specific effect on the disease?

Holy relics suffer from similar problems of authenticity and potency. Around 328 AD during a pilgrimage to Jerusalem, the future St Helena (mother of the Roman emperor Constantine) believed she had discovered the cross on which Jesus had been crucified. Cynics soon noted that so many supposedly genuine fragments of the True Cross had reached Europe that if they were all assembled in one place, there would have been enough wood to build several ships. The beautiful Sainte Chapelle in Paris was built by the pious King Louis IX to house what was alleged to be the True Crown of Thorns placed on the head of Jesus before his crucifixion. Louis had bought that rather dodgy relic, using up much of France's annual revenues in the process, from Baldwin II, son of the thuggish and usurping Emperor Baldwin I of Constantinople, who had ransacked the city during a crusade. There is no reason to suppose that either the True Cross or the True Crown are any more genuine than the Shroud of Turin, carbon-dated to around 1300 and recently shown to have had its authenticity strongly questioned at that time as a "patent example of clerical fraud".[184] Interestingly, some relics gain their alleged potency not by virtue of their original history but by merely having been in contact with the supposedly real thing, just like the homoeopathic notion that serially diluted solutions somehow retain a 'memory' of the original undiluted solution.

Prof. Duffin says that "the Vatican defines and diagnoses a miracle when the doctor is surprised". It also prefers that a recovery attributed to intercession by the putative saint should be 'instantaneous', though in practice, there's a bit of wiggle-room. I end this chapter, therefore with the case-history of an almost instantaneous cure that greatly surprised my non-psychiatric colleagues. Anna was a 35-year-old teacher. A year before I saw her, she suffered a straightforward lower leg fracture after a fall at home. There were no issues of compensation but her recovery was complicated and prolonged by a deep vein thrombosis in the injured leg. The fracture happened at a time when her marriage was breaking up and she naturally found the whole situation very distressing. When the plaster cast was removed, it took her a long time to regain even partial limb-movement. There were occasional short-lived improvements but when I was asked to see her in the orthopaedic ward, she was once more in bed. The injured leg, she told me, was paralysed and stiff. It wouldn't bend at all at the knee and only slightly at the hip. She was willing to talk about the marital problems but felt that they were in the past and she couldn't see how they could be related to her leg problem. She liked teaching (this was about 1968 when such affection for the profession was normal), wanted to get back to it and was suffering financially by not being able to do so.

Physical examination showed a classic type of hysterical or psychogenic paralysis. There was little muscle wasting, the knee jerks and other tendon reflexes were essentially normal and attempts to move the allegedly paralysed leg in any particular direction were met with vigorous resistance from the opposing muscle groups. ('Hysterical', in this context, is not a term of abuse and is discussed in more detail later. For the moment, let us simply say that it implies an essentially psychological mechanism with no corresponding physical abnormality of the relevant bits of the body, or the brain or of the nerves supplying the area in question.) When I asked her to try to bring her knee up and put it near her chin, she declared it impossible. The other leg was unaffected. At this stage, the cynical or puzzled reader might suggest two explanations. Perhaps Anna's stiff leg had some important symbolic meaning, hidden alike from her and me but possibly related (as posited by Freudian theory) to events in her childhood or to some ambivalence about work or divorce. Alternatively, given the fact that her muscles were obviously working perfectly well, perhaps there was some deliberate and devious mechanism at work. Perhaps she didn't really like teaching or was actually thinking about suing the surgeon or her ex-husband.

I can't tell you whether either of these explanations was anywhere near the truth (though I suspect that neither of them was) but I can tell you how I treated her paralysis with an unusual but logical mixture of cognitive and pharmacological techniques that would be administratively very difficult to arrange now but was followed by almost instant and lasting cure. Whatever the nature or explanation of Anna's condition, it evidently involved a genuine belief that her leg was stiff and could not bend in the normal way. One of the principles of cognitive-behavioural therapy is that the therapist must challenge incorrect or unhelpful 'maladaptive' beliefs and habits that are preventing the patient from achieving what both patient and therapist have agreed on as the goals of treatment. The other principle is that having jointly agreed and identified more appropriate habits of thinking and behaving, the therapist helps and encourages the patient to practise them until they become the new norm. I could not simply argue Anna into giving up her belief. The surgeons had been trying hard for many months to do that without success, though putting her in bed was probably not the best way of getting her to change her attitude. However, if I could even temporarily remove the unhelpful belief about her leg, it might be possible to show her that the limb could actually move and bend normally. Even with hypnosis, which I never mastered and to which not all patients are susceptible, it may be difficult to remove an isolated thought, especially in five minutes but it is possible to banish all thought quite easily by sending someone to sleep for a few minutes with a short-acting intravenous sedative. This I did, there and then, and while Anna was asleep, we easily bent her leg into the position that she had declared impossible only a few minutes before. When Anna woke up, the first thing she saw, a few inches from her eyes, was her knee. This state of affairs is called 'cognitive dissonance'. Anna could resolve it in two ways. She could either believe that what she was seeing was not actually her knee or she could accept that it was indeed her own knee and that therefore the belief that her leg could not bend must have been incorrect. Not surprisingly, she chose the second, more logical explanation.

Seizing the moment, I suggested that we ought to go for a little walk. Anna agreed and started walking but wanted to keep near the walls of the corridor to support herself in case she fell. I argued that doing so would only reinforce her belief that her leg was very weak, which was precisely what we were trying to change. So we walked up and down the middle of the corridor while I provided no more than a guiding hand on her arm. Occasionally she seemed about to fall and I had to stop the nurses from running to assist her. Within five minutes, Anna herself was running. She needed no further treatment and did not relapse. I think the main reason she did not relapse despite the long history was that whatever factors may have contributed to the onset of the paralysis, they no longer existed and there was therefore no real psychological need for it to continue. She had just got into inappropriate habits of thought and behaviour.

Since the elephant-joke fallacy could apply to this case as well as to CAM practitioners (and to the invocation of saints) I cannot be certain that my intervention specifically caused Anna's cure. She might have been about to get better anyway and my presence merely coincidental. She might also have responded in a general, placebo-ish, non-specific way to my admittedly impressive and even theatrical total treatment package, rather than being healed by the two specific components of it that I thought crucial. A particularly charismatic priest or CAM therapist might have overcome her initial inability to move her leg by strength of personality alone. However, I was using well-researched and well-validated psychological theories and a widely used sedative. I did not have to invoke mysterious forces as priests and homoeopaths do, medications of doubtful purity or efficacy like herbalists, or anatomical structures and pathways unknown to anatomical science like acupuncturists.

To one of Prof. Duffin's criticisms, incidentally, I plead partially guilty. She asks whether I realise that I am prejudiced "against the Catholic church and against religious belief in general". It is true that like many Europeans and most Danes and Swedes (and Einstein) I don't believe in a god who supposedly takes a close and personal interest in our individual welfare and I don't believe that sacred books are reliable and unambiguous guides to either history or morality. Whether my scepticism about the existence of god is absolute (atheism) or probabilistic (agnosticism) is irrelevant because in going about the ordinary business of life, both varieties of religious sceptic behave and think as if there is no god. However, I have tried in this book to examine some important and under-acknowledged drivers of religious belief and to help readers to understand why, like placebo effects, they can be so 'natural', powerful and comforting. I think I understand and respect placebo effects more than most people and therefore I think I also understand the particular appeal of the Catholic and High Anglican churches, so rich in symbolism, ritual, theatre and real, claimed or fabricated history. I like liturgical music and have sung motets, masses, passions and requiems in well-known choirs and cathedrals. (Incidentally, just as it is possible to be a popular and competent priest without having religious beliefs, several composers of the great requiems and masses were atheists, agnostics or vague in their beliefs, once unbelief no longer meant ostracism or worse. Those born in the 19th century include Berlioz, Brahms, Fauré, Janacek, Verdi and Vaughan-Williams. Beethoven was probably a deist.)

In psychiatry, we get to know our patients very well and I always made a point of asking mine about their religious beliefs because if they are important for the patient, they will probably be important for me to know about. I have successfully treated several clergymen, to whom I sometimes made my own position clear, if only to give them the option of receiving treatment from a fellow-believer if they preferred. A few years after his recovery, one of them invited me, in my psychiatric capacity, to his retirement dinner hosted by the then Archbishop of Canterbury at Lambeth Palace. It is partly because of these encounters that I became interested in the interactions and conflicts between their profession and mine.

Christianity no longer directly threatens the life and liberty of unbelievers but the 'poisonous enthusiasms' that used to be a feature of all major Christian denominations until the 19th century are now a particular hallmark of Roman Catholicism among the main Christian churches in Europe, as well as of Islam and the numerous derivative and post-colonial varieties of Protestantism in Third World countries and the USA. It is Catholicism, more than any other major Christian sect, that positively encourages the cults of Holy Relics, saints, miracles and intercessionary prayer. Its claims are more unequivocal and more startling and therefore more to be questioned but this book is not really aimed at true believers, or their shrines. My main focus is on trying to explain some aspects of the psychology of symptom relief to people who are not dogmatic believers, or are undecided, and to show how much the relief of symptoms through religious processes has in common with placebo and non-specific effects in medicine.

Nevertheless, just as I criticize some aspects of religion, I also feel an obligation to answer some of the criticisms of unbelievers that are regularly made by religious leaders, especially when they attack our morality or alleged lack of it. Catholicism has long claimed a large patch of moral high ground that several recent financial and sexual scandals have revealed as laughably unmerited. The former Pope Benedict XVI asked rhetorically: "How are we to explain the fact that people who regularly received the Lord's body and confessed their sins in the sacrament of penance, have offended in this way? It remains a mystery".[185] It is no mystery to most people. There were many popes whose sexual habits before and after election appear rather tacky even by today's more relaxed standards. Yet those papal voluptuaries, embezzlers and fornicators (with both sexes) not only 'regularly received the Lord's body and confessed their sins' but were supposedly elected with God's personal guidance in solemn conclaves of the Vatican's most senior clerics. Of more recent Vatican moral failures, the fact that Pius XII automatically excommunicated every Communist in 1948 but did not excommunicate a single Nazi during or after the war stands out. Many of the communists were probably unbelievers but there was no shortage of practising Catholic Nazis in Germany and Austria, and among their equivalents elsewhere in occupied Europe.

Almost every day, I pass the bridge in London under which Roberto Calvi was murdered in 1982. He was known as 'God's Banker' because of his close links with the Vatican. Another financial intimate of Popes, Michele Sindona, was poisoned in his prison cell, Borgia-style, with cyanide-enriched coffee. The Vatican isn't included in Transparency International's Index of Corruption but it swims in an Italian sea and for all its *dolce vita,* Italy – historically not just Catholic but almost Protestant-free - is the most corrupt country in Western Europe. In 2023, it was the 42nd among the 180 countries in Transparency International's league (1st = best) and scored 56 on a scale from 0 ("highly corrupt") to 100 ("very clean"). It is even more corrupt than the other historically Catholic countries at the bottom of the EU transparency league – Spain, Malta and Slovakia. Only Greece and Romania are worse.[186] Of the top ten least corrupt countries, all but one are historically Protestant and now have large proportions of the unbelieving or indifferent. The non-Protestant exception is Singapore, which is largely Confucian or Buddhist and determinedly secular.

It is that long history of corruption in Italian Catholicism and Italian society that causes me to have a few doubts about the conclusions of the *Consulta Medica.* We can have little faith in supposedly miraculous cancer cures that were proclaimed before the late 19th century, when microscopic examination of diseased human tissues began to make histological diagnosis increasingly reliable. Many other incapacitating or potentially lethal conditions could not be accurately diagnosed until the following century and misdiagnosis must have been common but even when diagnosis became a more precise science, I suspect that the show had to go on and the miracles had to keep coming. How could the Vatican explain to the faithful that God had stopped performing the medical miracles that so distinguish it from the Church of England? Is it unreasonable to wonder whether some diagnostic arm-twisting or self-censorship took place?

My suspicions are strengthened by the massive and well-documented financial corruption in the saint-making process revealed by the Italian journalist Gianluigi Nuzzi. Dioceses that put forward candidates for canonisation and beatification have to finance the proceedings with sums that average half a million Euros and each case is overseen by an official called a Postulator. A proportion of any money that remains is supposed to go to the Fund for the Causes of the Poor, intended for dioceses that find it difficult to finance a process but it was discovered that this fund remained suspiciously small and stagnant. The 'Congregation for the Causes of Saints' initially did everything it could to obstruct COSEA, the independent commission belatedly appointed by Pope Francis to look into the financial affairs of the Vatican. Eventually, the Congregation's accounts were frozen. It emerged that there were a couple of almost full-time Postulators who each handled 90 cases compared with an average of 5 - 6 for the other 400+ Postulators. One of them was found to have nearly a million Euros in his blocked accounts. Nepotism and inflated consultancy fees, combined with an absence of accounting and the offer by one Postulator "to conduct an investigation even before opening a canonization process, on the condition that he receive an initial payment of 40,000 Euros", as well as the unprecedented increase in saint-production, make accusations of fraud and racketeering difficult to avoid.[187] Under Norm 27(c) of the 'New [1983] Laws for the Causes of Saints', the Postulator may add documents of his own before the final submission. Cardinal Giovanni Becciu, sentenced in 2023 by the Vatican to five years in prison for embezzlement, had been the Prefect of the Dicastery (previously the Congregation) of the Causes of Saints from 2018 until his 'resignation under duress' in 2020. The function of the Dicastery (thanks again, Wikipedia) is to oversee "the complex process that leads to the canonization of saints, passing through the steps of a declaration of 'heroic virtues' and beatification. After preparing a case, including the approval of miracles, the case is presented to the Pope, who decides whether or not to proceed with beatification or canonization". In November 2024, Dr Sergio Alfieri, who had recently operated on Pope Francis, was "charged with fraud in connection with allegedly fake records of operations he never performed ... [claiming] that he was in the operating theatre when he was, at times, hundreds of miles away. ... Alfieri, who "sits on the board of the Gemelli Hospital Foundation and the Vatican Health Commission, denies any wrongdoing."[188]

Neither individual Catholics nor individual priests are responsible for the sins of the Vatican. Many parishioners and quite a few priests privately reject large parts of Catholic doctrine, notably where it involves contraception. Precisely because they embody and promote tradition and familiar ritual, religions tend to resist change but the history of Catholicism is particularly rich in last-ditch defences of the indefensible, from opposing democratisation and freedom of conscience to opposing gas-lighting and railways. (Pope Gregory XVI punned that railways were not *chemins de fer* (iron roads) but *chemins d'enfer* (roads to hell). Unlike the Church of England, it rarely apologises for its past sins of omission and commission. As theologian and historian Joseph Hoffmann wrote:

> "Religion alone seems able to convince ordinary people that there is no point at which abuses and sins become definitive and not exceptional: imagine judging a serial rapist by saying that he's simply failing to live up to his ideals and that, for all appearances, he's really a very nice chap."[189]

What are we to make of lectures on morality and the sanctity of life from the spiritual heirs of the Inquisition and the Borgia Popes?

Chapter 12
"That placebo made me feel really ill!"
Harmful nocebo effects in religion and medicine

"Placebo Controls, Exorcisms and the Devil"[190] was arguably the most unusual paper published by Prof Kaptchuk and his Harvard colleagues and it describes the application of placebo-controlled clinical trial principles five centuries ago. The Renaissance may not have been as radical as the Enlightenment but it produced a good crop of sceptics. Unfortunately, in an age when religion still permeated every waking moment, their focus was mostly theological and several of the most prominent sceptics died a heretic's death. Rather than testing the effectiveness of medical treatments, the trial exhumed by the Harvard team tested claims that theologians could reliably detect possession by the offspring or assistants of the Devil – incubi, succubi and assorted demons.

The Renaissance also gave rise to the Protestant Reformation and in France, as in Europe more generally, to ferocious wars of religion between Catholics and the French Protestants – the Huguenots. They are depressingly similar to the wars of religion between Sunni and Shia Muslims, currently tearing apart the Islamic world and spilling over into the streets of countries in which the importance of religion has been steadily declining. After the 1572 St Bartholomew's Day massacre of prominent Huguenots visiting Paris for a controversial royal wedding (the pious and perennially gloomy Philip II of Spain was said to have "laughed for the only time on record" on hearing of it) there was an uneasy peace. Henri IV, the Huguenot king, converted to Catholicism ("Paris is worth a Mass") and both brands of Christianity coexisted unhappily under Henri's Edict of Nantes until Louis XIV revoked it a century later. The unhappy coexistence occurred during several centuries of witch-hunting in Europe and North America and the closely related phenomenon of demonic possession. Mass possession and its modern equivalents are covered in more detail in the next chapter. This one looks at the ways in which some more thoughtful French Catholics used the principles of the placebo-controlled trial to detect false accusations by Catholic zealots who used claims of demonic possession as a weapon in the war against Protestantism. It also describes the ways in which the powerful placebo and non-specific processes that can make people feel very much better can also make them feel very much worse.

Although most allegations of demonic possession reflected popular religious beliefs of an age that regarded Beelzebub and his satanic legions as a very real presence in everyday life (even a century later, "Most men and women in…Britain still lived in a world of magic, in which God and the devil intervened daily, a world of witches, fairies and charms.")[191] some allegations were attempts to remove enemies or competitors by falsely accusing them of being possessed. As Kaptchuk and his colleagues explain:

> "[T]his power to cast out the devil and his confederates became a persuasive tool for demonstrating apostolic authority. This was especially the case for Catholics who were more comfortable with miraculous displays. These Counter-Reformation exorcisms depended on the 'common knowledge' that demons could not tolerate direct divine contact (e.g. contact with holy water, consecrated wafer or readings from the Latin scriptures). Such exposures caused the demons to writhe in pain and flee the body with a consequent 'cure' for the possession victim. Not surprisingly, Catholic priests would urge devils to testify to their fondness of Protestants and fear of Rome".

Exorcisms were often major public events and an opportunity for amusement as well as for theological and spiritual struggle. "In bawdy relief, the possessed demoniacs provided entertainment with erotic ditties, lewd gestures, wild gyrations, hideous faces and wild, shrieking animal roars. Breathtaking feats of physical prowess were exhibited in the violent wrestling between teams of strongmen and newly invigorated demoniacs. Audiences could reach 20,000". We shall see how equally remarkable "feats of physical prowess" can be induced by hypnosis.

Not everyone welcomed these theological circuses. Some in the French Catholic hierarchy had enough sense to realise that the typically anti-Huguenot atmosphere damaged France's fragile social cohesion. "Protestants, who generally had an anti-magical critique of Catholicism, were suspicious and easily discounted these superstitious events ... Some argued that possessed victims (who were overwhelmingly women) probably had severe illnesses, were coerced by zealot preachers or simply gave false testimony." In a response to one alleged possession that could easily have fanned the sectarian flames, Catholic sceptics devised a "trick trial" that, while not questioning the existence of demons, at least questioned the diagnostic criteria for demonic possession. The politico-religious stakes were high because the ink on the Edict of Nantes was barely dry when some anti-Huguenot priests were called to exorcise a young Catholic woman. She was supposedly possessed by Beelzebub himself who, according to the priests, repeatedly testified that "all the Huguenots belonged to him".

Fearing the consequences, Henri IV formed a hasty commission very similar to the one formed two centuries later by his successor Louis XVI to investigate Anton Mesmer and his 'animal magnetism'. After removing the poor woman from the charged public atmosphere, they tested the diagnostic claims by repeatedly giving her 'genuine' holy water without telling her it was holy. Nothing happened. No Protestant demons emerged spewing anti-Catholic sentiments. They then did a 'crossover' trial of the kind described in Chapter 6 that involved "giving her ordinary water poured from a special flask known to be only used for holy water", following which "she contorted in pain". Then, "When an ordinary piece of iron was taken out of its ornate enclosure and presented to the young woman as a relic of the true cross, she fell to the ground tormented. Priests read to the women a Latin text, misinforming her that it was the Holy Scripture. In actuality, it was Virgil's *Aeneid*, and she nonetheless squirmed in agony." These were essentially nocebo effects, mediated by purely psychological mechanisms – chiefly suggestion and expectation - in the same way that placebo effects are.

The first recorded mention of a controlled trial – though not randomized or using a placebo and with only two 'patients' – actually predates this Reformation example by a couple of thousand years, appearing in the Old Testament.[192] Like much of the Old Testament, it is also fictional but it was allegedly a trial of the effectiveness of two gods: Jehovah (or Yahwe) the god of ancient Israel and Baal, the god of a neighbouring kingdom. The prophet Elijah challenged the priests of Baal to get their god to light a fire beneath a sacrificial animal. When their prayers were unanswered, Elijah called on Jehovah to do the job properly, which he did even though Elijah had previously poured water on the firewood. The priests of Baal did not immediately convert to Judaism because Elijah had them all killed.

Nearly all drugs can cause side-effects or, to use the increasingly favoured term, 'adverse effects' (AEs). Surprisingly, placebos sometimes produce as many AEs (i.e. nocebo effects) as active drugs. Some drug AEs are serious and life-threatening and treatment decisions always involve balancing the likely benefits of treatment against the likely harms. 'Do no harm' is a counsel of perfection and in an imperfect world, the best that physicians and surgeons can do is to keep the level of harm as low as possible. Placebo-controlled trials generally measure AEs in both active and placebo groups but nocebo effects are so common that if AEs are found only in the active group, there is probably something wrong with the trial. For drugs with few AEs, there may be no difference between active and placebo groups. For example, in a trial involving fewer than a hundred patients and a drug like ordinary penicillin, whose sole important AE is an allergic reaction affecting less than 1% of patients, there may well be no allergic patients among the 50 in the active group. Nocebo effects occurring in the placebo group are usually minor and transient, as are many AEs with a pharmacological basis but some 'side effects' are surprisingly severe for pills or potions that have no pharmacologically active ingredients. In patients assigned to placebo groups, the perceived AEs are sufficiently severe that as many as 26% discontinue the placebos.[193] Furthermore, all these unpleasant, harmful effects can be reduced or increased in the same way that beneficial placebo effects can be reduced or increased - by variations in the 'sales technique' such as gold-plating or colouring the placebo pills, increasing their size or dose, or replacing placebo pills with placebo injections. When patients know they are definitely receiving a placebo tablet, they experience far fewer AEs than when they receive a tablet that they know could be either a placebo or an active drug.[194]

One common and clinically important factor that is guaranteed to increase nocebo effects is to give patients detailed information about every side effect that their (genuine) medicines might cause – a practice almost unknown when I qualified but now a mandatory feature of dispensing. When patients thought they were receiving a placebo but were actually given a common anti-migraine drug that can certainly cause AEs, some of them serious, they reported no more AEs than patients who received the active drug but thought they were receiving the placebo. Conversely, when the same drug was labelled with its correct name, its analgesic effect increased by 50%, highlighting the similarity and interdependence of both placebo and nocebo effects.[195]

In everyday life, the equivalents of nocebo effects are seen in the many people who strongly believe that they are harmed by things that, as judged by more elaborate and systematic versions of Henri IV's blinded substitution tests, actually have no physical effects at all. One large group of this kind are the people who believe that electromagnetic radiation from power lines and wi-fi equipment is making them ill. Their condition is common enough to have its own impressive name and acronym - Idiopathic Environmental Intolerance Attributed to Electromagnetic Fields (IEI-EMF). If the attribution were correct, it would have important implications for the design and siting of power lines and so it has been studied. While studies funded or initiated by power companies might be suspect or fraudulent (as some infamous studies sponsored by tobacco companies most certainly were) there is no shortage of academics without any obvious axe to grind – other than the desire to contribute to the sum of knowledge – who are keen to investigate the matter impartially. Repeated investigations have shown that although the sufferers from IEI-EMF firmly believe that they can reliably detect the presence of electromagnetic radiation, as the exorcists and exorcees of Renaissance France believed that they could reliably detect the presence of demons, they were unable to manage it more than the 50% of the time that chance would have predicted when they were tested under blind conditions.[196] "At present, there is no reliable evidence to suggest that people with IEI-EMF experience unusual physiological reactions as a result of exposure to EMF. This supports suggestions that EMF is not the main cause of their ill health".[197] Since one of the common complaints was that electromagnetic radiation adversely affected their sleep, this review of the literature includes some studies that made electro-encephalographic (EEG) recordings during sleep when the current was on or off. The patients were not only unaware of their true state of exposure to the radiation: they were unaware of anything at all while they were asleep. When their sleeping EEG tracings were compared, no differences in their brain-waves were found. "[W]orry about a modern technology increases the chances of someone attributing symptoms to it" and similar problems have been wrongly attributed to a more recent and controversial feature of our landscape. "[For] wind turbines, there is already some evidence that a nocebo effect can explain the attributed symptoms". Not surprisingly, "social factors, including media reporting and interaction with lobby groups can increase symptom reporting".[198]

Since the beginning of the Industrial Revolution, almost every new technological development has been similarly accused of damaging health, not in obvious and direct ways such as railway and motor accidents, electric shocks or internet addiction but through mysterious, invisible and unmeasurable emanations. In their turn, radio waves, flying machines and x-rays were all put in the same pillory as IEI-EMF and wind turbines and the exponential growth of technology and inventions means that there will be plenty of new imagined threats to join them. Each one is an example of the power of belief, meaning and nocebo effects to create symptoms: and of the power of both medical and religious placebo effects to remove them.

Chapter 13
The madness of crowds
Mass and individual hysteria from the Devils of Loudun to
Charcot's Paris

There are two reasons why the story of Anna and her paralysed leg, in Chapter 11, is relevant to a discussion of placebo effects. It shows that individual cases involving 'hysterical' symptoms can sometimes explain sudden cures and it also shows that severe hysterical or psychogenic disorders can occur in very ordinary and unremarkable people. *Epidemics* of hysterical disorder can also affect 'ordinary' people and they still happen, though modern epidemics are often much less dramatic than the older ones. (Delayed trigger warning: I discuss the re-naming of 'hysteria' shortly.) They used to be a lot commoner and instead of being wrongly attributed to viruses, gases or toxins as they often are today, they were usually seen until two or three centuries ago as the work of The Devil and thought of as 'possession', an even more worrying manifestation of Satan's power than the individual cases just described. This chapter is about some of those older epidemics and the evolution of attitudes to hysteria since then.

Around 1730 in Paris, an outbreak of religious convulsions occurred in the vicinity of the church of St Médard, where healing miracles were attributed to an ascetic and good-looking young cleric with a taste for self-flagellation, who had recently died. Some of his followers also flagellated themselves and even, it is said, had themselves briefly crucified. (Being crucified with real nails – though not to the point of death – is still a regular event in the Philippines during Holy Week.) These *'convulsionnaires'* seem to have had varying motives, some seeking relief from illnesses and others seeking religious ecstasy, but they became such a public nuisance that they were suppressed. Several were sent to the Bastille and the cemetery of St Médard was closed to the public. They were also a political nuisance because many were members of a dissident and puritanical Catholic sect called Jansenists. The nuns of the main Jansenist convent at Port Royal des Champs had earlier been forcibly dispersed and their buildings were demolished soon afterwards.

A contemporary reporter, while declaring that "among the convulsionists there were occasionally to be found persons of respectable standing" added significantly: "But it must be confessed that in general, God has chosen the convulsionists among the common people; that they were chiefly young children, especially girls; that almost all of them had lived till then in ignorance and obscurity; that several of them were deformed, and some, in their natural state, even exhibited imbecility. Of such, for the most part, it was that God made choice, to show forth to us His power." Equally unsurprising is that among those seeking relief from illness, "The greater number are cases of paralysis, usually of one entire side of the body", which is rather typical of hysterical paralyses[199], hemiplegia (unilateral paralysis) due to strokes being very uncommon in the young.

I'm not using these descriptions as a put-down of women. The greater occurrence of mass and individual hysteria in women (at least in peacetime) does not reflect any inherent, constitutional weakness or inferiority of women. Psychiatric opinion generally holds that hysterical symptoms are more likely in any group who are relatively restricted by custom or status in their ability to ventilate anger or domestic distress directly. Culturally, this has been the lot of most women throughout history. It still is their lot in most of the world and things have changed only recently in developed countries where women have real rights (as opposed to theoretical ones) increasingly similar to those of men. For different reasons, both male and female members of groups such as children, people with low IQ, immigrants who have not acculturated to the host country (especially if they cannot communicate easily with the local health professionals) may also have difficulty in disclosing their true feelings, which may therefore be expressed, though not in a fully conscious way, as pain, paralysis, vomiting, convulsions or even coma. Pain is now the commonest expression of poorly-articulated discontents and its uncomprehending sufferers stretch the capacity of every GP surgery, most out-patient clinics and several in-patient units.

An earlier and better-known example of mass possession and religious hysteria occurred in the town of Loudun, not far from Tours in western France. It is better known because Aldous Huxley described it in his book, *The Devils of Loudun,* that was used by John Whiting and Ken Russell to make a play and a film respectively, both called *The Devils.* It occurred in the mid-17th century when the European and early American obsession with witchcraft was reaching the last of its several peaks. The Ken Russell film, for which the young Derek Jarman did some of his first cinema work, portrays vomiting, writhing, shrieking, and convulsing nuns, sometimes shouting unholy obscenities or speaking in tongues (i.e. speaking nonsense) for good measure.

If you think this sort of thing doesn't happen in modern, Western societies, you're mistaken. Matt Taibbi, a reporter for *Rolling Stone* magazine and later its editor, reported undercover on a weekend of demon-related activities run by an American Evangelical pastor called Fortenberry.

"'In the name of Jesus, I cast out the demon of incest! In the name of Jesus, I cast out the demon of sexual abuse!' ... I was beginning to think the Deliverance was going to be a bust. But then it started. Wails and cries from the audience. To my left, a young black man started writhing around in his seat. In front of me and to my right, another young black man ... started wailing and clutching his head. 'In the name of Jesus,' continued Fortenberry, 'I cast out the demon of astrology!' Coughing and spitting noises. Behind me, a bald white man started to wheeze and gurgle [and] began power-puking into his paper baggie. I couldn't see if any actual vomitus came out, but he made real hurling and retching noises.

Now the women began to pipe in ... and ... if you've ever watched *The Houston 560* or any other gangbang porn movie, that's what it sounded like, only the sounds were far more intense. It was not difficult to figure out where the energy was coming from on that side of the room. Some of the husbands glanced nervously over in the direction of their wives. 'In the name of Jesus Christ, I cast out the demon of cancer!' said Fortenberry. 'Oooh! Unnh! Unnnnnh!' wailed a woman in the front row. 'Bleeech!' puked the bald man behind me. Within about a minute after that, the whole chapel erupted in pandemonium. About half the men and three-fourths of the women were writhing around and either play-puking or screaming.

Once you've made a journey like this -- once you've gone this far -- you are beyond suggestible ... you've left behind the mental process that a person would need to form an independent opinion about such things. You make this journey precisely to experience the ecstasy of beating to the same big gristly heart with a roomful of like-minded folks. Once you reach that place with them, you're thinking with muscles, not neurons."[200]

Induced or self-induced quasi-hypnotic states are sometimes associated with visions and other phenomena typical of powerful religious experiences. Many saints (especially but not exclusively female saints) were reported to have behaved in ways suggestive of popular conceptions of hypnotic trances, though so-called 'trance' states are probably not a specific, hypnotic phenomenon. They can also occur in the absence of attempts at hypnosis.

In this chapter and one or two preceding ones, I've used a rather loaded word – hysteria – that will make some people bristle. It's widely regarded in psychiatry as old-fashioned, stigmatizing and Not Politically Correct. We are supposed to use terms like 'conversion disorder' or 'somatisation disorder' for individual cases and 'mass psychogenic (or sociogenic) illness' for the kind that affects groups of people. People who are interested in the history of psychiatry or the history of medicine in general know that something called 'hysteria' was once common and that whatever it was, women got it much more often than men. They may have seen old black and white photographs of the 19th century Parisian neurologist Jean-Martin Charcot 'demonstrating' female hysterics, who are wearing long Victorian skirts and standing in extraordinary postures. Medical students are presumably still taught that the term comes from the Greek word for the womb because hysteria was once believed to be due to the uterus breaking loose and wandering through the body, leaving a selection of tiresome, Eve-ish dysfunctions in its wake. We are supposed to have abandoned such absurd and paternalistic theories a long time ago but it takes more than a bare half-century of evidence-based medicine and a slightly longer period of female emancipation to shake off a fine old bit of medical mythology; especially one that enabled men to feel superior to women. We may not hear so much about hysteria these days but that doesn't mean that the behaviour and the syndromes that attracted a 'hysterical' label in the late 19th and early 20th centuries have gone away. It may have been re-labelled as part of the campaign to de-stigmatise mental disorders but it is still common and like all medical conditions, it varies considerably in severity.

Journalists, like ordinary people, still use words like 'hysteria' and 'hysterical' to describe any reaction or behaviour that they deem to be 'excessive' or 'too emotional'. They may also use it to mean 'un-British' in the sense of not showing enough of that stiff upper-lip that is still an important part of our national self-image, though perhaps a diminishing one. "Hysteria", says the feminist historian Elaine Showalter "is the opposite of the cherished national trait of irony". She quotes two self-confident Victorian British alienists who believed that: "... the Latin races are much more prone to hysteria than are those who come of Teutonic stock" and another who wrote: "The Gallic nature seems to be of less enduring stability than the Saxon and is more liable to exhibit exalted hysterical manifestations".[201] You can see how the term became un-PC.

To doctors, hysteria used to mean conditions, especially conditions with mainly neurological manifestations such as paralysis or loss of sensation, that didn't appear to have any obvious physical cause. The typical hysteric was a woman complaining that she had lost the use of one or more limbs or of her sight or voice, often quite suddenly. Even to use a word like 'complaining' could be misleading because a common feature of these disabilities was that the women concerned often seemed to be not very worried about them. They might even smile while describing them. This *belle indifférence*, as it is called, was thought to be almost diagnostic of hysteria because surely any normal woman – and certainly any normal man – would be rather worried if their right arm suddenly seized up. No doubt about it; these women were up to their old Eve-ish tricks again and making life needlessly difficult for their doctors. Who, as it happened, were nearly all men. It didn't help matters that Freud devoted much of his early writing to hysteria, linking it with the usual causative suspects from murky childhoods, though at least he didn't make the mistake of thinking that hysteria couldn't happen in men. It's just that nearly all the allegedly hysterical patients he wrote about were women.

Feminists have mixed feelings about all these psychoanalytical put-downs of women from overwhelmingly male clinicians. Initially, if feminists criticised psychoanalysis at all, it was for its stereotyping of women as hopelessly emotional and impractical creatures at heart, thus giving aid and comfort to the persistent view in some quarters that women are constitutionally unsuited to the task of running a country or even of voting for its parliamentary representatives. Women's suffrage is less than a hundred years old in most countries, reaching France, Italy and Switzerland only after WW2. Women doctors stopped being in a small minority in Britain only during my lifetime.

If you can't find a physical cause for a prominent or disabling symptom, it is natural to wonder whether the cause might be psychological or, in the currently preferred locutions, psychogenic or sociogenic. Often, this is a reasonable train of thought, especially if the symptom's first appearance happened to coincide with some significant stress, but there are potential diagnostic hazards with such formulations. The first is the old but still very sound maxim that absence of evidence is not evidence of absence. With ever more sensitive and efficient diagnostic techniques, we are less likely to miss the early stages of serious disease but it still happens. The ability of some early cancers to produce weird and generalised neurological or hormonal disturbances far away from the site of the tumour is well documented. Sometimes, cancers that are too small to show up on scans or x-rays produce chemicals or hormones that can affect distant organs but even today, the earliest stages of a disease are often, almost by definition, the most difficult to detect and confirm. Here are two examples that could still occur today; and remember that the colourful Conservative MP, ex-minister and Pepys-like diarist Alan Clark died as recently as 1999 from a brain tumour that was originally thought to be something else.

As a very junior doctor, I once looked after a young married woman who had quite suddenly developed profound weakness of both legs. The neurological signs were unusual and inconsistent and her blood tests were virtually normal. She had experienced a few stresses recently but what made everyone think that this mysterious paralysis was probably 'hysterical' was that she remained cheerful and quite often actually *smiled*. I was asked to demonstrate her to the medical students as a classic case of hysterical paralysis with classic *belle indifférence*. Spinal x-rays had been reported as normal but when the films were being reviewed, a sharp-eyed radiologist thought that there was a very faint shadow that shouldn't have been there. After half a pint of pus was removed from a sneaky little abscess near her lumbar spine, she very quickly got better. The smile and the cheerfulness had meant only that she was the sort of person who wasn't easily depressed and who had a touching faith in doctors. In any case, even in the 1960s, people in their twenties had probably got used to thinking that to die young from acute illness was quite rare, unlike previous generations.

Another 'hysterical' patient was transferred to the psychiatric ward after the surgeons had failed to find a cause for her persistent vomiting. She too had experienced a few recent problems. They were actually pretty mundane and trivial ones but two and two were dutifully made to equal five. Surgeons used not to be famous for the thoroughness of their pre-operative examinations, though brain tumours are well recognised as one of the less common causes of persistent vomiting. Fortunately, junior psychiatrists are expected to know a bit of neurology and our examination was better than theirs. An ultra-sound brain scan – all we had in those days – was either normal or hadn't been done but simple ophthalmoscopic examination alerted us to the presence of a tumour.

The fact that both these patients were women was probably significant, for men with puzzling symptoms are much less likely to be suspected or accused of having an underlying 'psychological' cause. It's still apparently acceptable to pat women on the head and attribute their problem to 'nerves', with the implication of some personal weakness or of some generalised feminine predisposition. That's one reason why women receive most of the prescriptions for antidepressants and tranquillisers. Men often don't like receiving such suggestions from doctors and doctors often don't like making them to men. We are sometimes allowed to suggest that a physical symptom may be due to 'stress', which shifts the blame from the patient to the situation, or to the person who is supposed to have caused the stress but even that can be unwelcome to men who are supposed to thrive on stress, especially military men. Incidentally, exactly the same stress can produce completely different symptoms in different people. One of my dermatology teachers gave us the example of bus passengers reacting to a collision, shaken but not seriously injured. One vomits, another rushes to empty bladder or bowels. Alternatively, they might faint, develop a psychogenic paralysis or (the example that interested him) come out in a rash.

Although an early 19th century French physician famously said that men couldn't be hysterical because they had no uterus, classic hysterical symptoms had been recorded in men for centuries. Some physicians tried to square the circle by suggesting that such men were effeminate (read: homosexual) and therefore probably had a tiny womblet floating around somewhere. Others just came up with different names for the same condition. When soldiers who had fought in the American Civil War presented with strange symptoms, the term 'Soldiers Heart' was used. In the First World War, 'shell shock' was the alleged cause of classic hysterical paralyses as well as vaguer and more subjective complaints like headaches, loss of memory, poor sleep and whatever word men used then instead of 'depression'. Physicians were not only very reluctant to apply the term hysteria to male patients: they were also reluctant to mention their male hysterics in the medical journals. Showalter relates that the American neurologist Weir Mitchell wrote about a man with classic hysterical symptoms whom he followed up for nearly thirty years. The patient even willed his body for autopsy, though no brain lesion was found. Yet the account remained unread in Mitchell's papers until recently and although Charcot described a series of male hysterics, his paper was only translated into English barely three decades ago.

Once upon a time, there was a condition called neurasthenia. It was very common in the second half of the 19th century. It was also called American Nervousness or Nervous Exhaustion (perhaps even abbreviated in medical notes to 'N.E.'). Middle class and educated women were the main victims and their main complaints were weakness and fatigue. One fashionable treatment involved complete bed rest for several weeks without even books to read. Neurasthenia also covered much of what we now call 'depression' – a term not much used then. Its predilection for the middle classes is perhaps not difficult to explain.

Proletarian housewives or female manual workers complaining of generalised weakness would probably get little sympathy from husbands or employers. Accordingly, their hysterical symptoms tended to be more dramatic and more like known illnesses. Middle class women, in contrast, might not want to be associated with the mainly lower class 'grand hysterics' who populated Charcot's domain, so weakness and fatigue were probably more acceptable symptoms. Their servants would manage the household tasks allotted to them by the reclining patient but both types of disorder were seen in all social classes.

None of this is meant to imply that all hysterical conditions are fabricated, voluntary or 'imaginary' and still less that these conditions, whatever their ultimate cause, are therefore trivial or risible. However, if we exclude out-and-out malingering, we are probably dealing with a spectrum of awareness ranging from partial insight to a complete lack of it. In my experience, malingering has been rare, though it is probably less rare among front-line soldiers, especially conscripts. (Working in a quasi-military Veterans' hospital in Australia in 1970, I saw a 20-year old conscript who had shot his thumb off with a rifle to avoid being sent to Viet-Nam. He was a country boy of borderline low IQ and what seemed to have motivated him was not cowardice but annoyance at being taken away from a job with animals and prospects that a kindly farmer had given him.) However, according to a very well-placed and politically rather left-ish NHS doctor who specialised in assessing disability claims, malingering and exaggeration are extremely common in people seeking long-term sickness benefits. "When I first started working with them", she told me on strict conditions of anonymity, "I expected that no more than a third would be simulating or exaggerating their disability. After a few months, I had upped that to two thirds". In any case, when it comes to treatment, insight may not matter too much. 'Explaining' hysterical symptoms can be an interesting pseudo-intellectual pastime, especially for Freudians but this is one of those areas where relief without explanation really is better than explanation without relief. Here are a couple of case histories that show how profound mental, physical and behavioural changes can be caused by purely psychological, personality and social factors. The importance and relevance of these accounts is, firstly, that the same factors that can make people feel ill can also, in a different setting, make them feel well; and secondly, that similar processes underlie many cases of religious healing.

Case History 1.

An English woman in her fifties was admitted to hospital after suddenly becoming comatose. She didn't speak or respond to questions or move her limbs, even in response to painful stimuli, although she was still breathing normally. It was soon clear that this was almost certainly a psychogenic, hysterical coma because although all four limbs appeared to be limp and paralysed, the paralysis was selective. If I lifted an arm and released it, the arm fell back limply onto the bed or onto her chest but if the arm was released from a position where gravity would make it fall onto her face, it always veered away at the last moment. The muteness meant that we could not ask her what this behaviour might signify or symbolise but it first appeared shortly after her son had set a date for emigrating to Australia. She recovered in a few days without anything in the way of medical or psychiatric treatment, so the precise psychological mechanism remained even more speculative than usual, though the traumatic event was obvious enough. It may be the insidious influence of Freudian ideology, incidentally, that makes many quite literate people pronounce the word 'trauma' (*traw*'ma, as in 'straw' or 'author', from the Greek word for a physical or psychological wound) as if it were derived from the German word for a dream - *traum* – and pronounced *trow*'ma as in 'how' or 'cow'.

Case History 2.

A much more complicated patient, who also improved without any overt interpretation, explanation or acceptance of underlying psychological or emotional processes, was a fourteen-year old boy with trichotillomania – patchy baldness caused by pulling out his hair. Because the idea that teenage or younger children might be doing this seems weird, many cases are initially misdiagnosed as the skin disease alopecia and referred to a dermatologist, though the appearance of the hair and skin in true alopecia is quite different. Hair-pulling is often resistant to treatment and this boy needed to wear a wig by the time we saw him. We strongly suspected that there were serious problems at home but we had nothing specific to go on. Both the boy and his parents insisted that they were just an ordinary happy family and that, of course, the doctors must be wrong about the cause of the baldness. After several weeks without progress, we decided to try an ether abreaction.

The original idea behind abreaction was that by helping patients to understand and relive the traumatic experience that had allegedly caused the condition, the symptoms could be made to go away. It was used quite successfully in the Second World War for battle neurosis (i.e.

psychogenic symptoms such as paralysis) but it soon turned out that provided the soldiers were able to release a lot of emotion, they usually got better whether they emoted about a messy recent battle scene or about something completely unconnected with the War. In other words, the effect was rather non-specific. Sub-anaesthetic doses of anaesthetic drugs like ether or short-acting intravenous barbiturates were often used to help patients talk more freely. (The KGB was not the only organisation to use that effect on spies and political prisoners.) When taken in small doses, ether and barbiturates can release inhibitions, rather like alcohol. 'Ether frolics' and their laughing-gas equivalents were a popular early 19th century manifestation of recreational drug use and were the equivalent of glue-sniffing, though in those days, it was a middle-class and grown-up activity. Not at all like the barely pubescent underclass glue-heads of recent times.

After a few lungfuls of ether, the boy started talking – or rather, screaming. It wasn't easy to understand what he was saying but phrases like 'Don't hit her' were clear enough. Our suspicions about his family life seemed vindicated but when he emerged from the ether haze, blandness and denial quickly returned. He said he couldn't remember much about the procedure, which was probably true, since amnesia is usually the sign of a good abreaction. We suggested that the things he had said under the influence of ether indicated that all was not well at home. Not so, he insisted. Everything was just fine. Was his father ever violent to his mother? No, never. Not even hardly ever. Fortunately, since the procedure wasn't done very often, the clinic sister had suggested that we should record the abreaction as a teaching aid. In that paternalistic and deferential era, it was not thought necessary to seek the patient's consent. We played it back to him, screams and all. Nothing was said but he looked thoughtful. I don't know what went through his mind but the hair-pulling stopped and didn't return.

I don't find it difficult to believe that in a religious culture and setting, patients can sometimes make equally complete recoveries from incapacitating illnesses with a purely psychological cause under the care of priests, especially charismatic ones. That is what procedures like exorcism involve and it might reflect spontaneous recovery, as in Case 1, or the release of very powerful emotions, as in Case 2. However, failed abreactions – i.e. when no emotion or useful information emerges or the symptoms persist – usually leave patients no worse than they were before the procedure. Exorcism may simply replace one unhelpful set of beliefs with another.

Chapter 14
Therapeutic nationalism: bad for truth.
Medical research should put out fewer flags

It is natural that people tend to have more faith in doctors and treatments coming from their own cultural group and sometimes less faith in those that don't. We have already seen how placebo medicines and procedures (and CAM) vary considerably between cultures but nationalism also affects more orthodox medicine and its practitioners. I begin with the story of the cancer 'multitherapy' developed by the Italian Dr Luigi Di Bella in the late 1980s. Dr Di Bella (1912-2003) was not only a doctor but also a professor of physiology at the ancient University of Modena, founded in 1175. A search of PubMed indicates that for much of his career, he published uncontroversial papers on a range of physiological topics but he eventually focused on the effects on various cancers of the naturally occurring hormone melatonin and of several other drugs. I myself was prescribing one of these other drugs, octreotide, for equally 'off-label'[202] but entirely different reasons (I fortuitously discovered that it is the best drug for controlling diarrhoea and vomiting during rapid opiate withdrawal)[203, 204, 205] and so I kept encountering Di Bella's name and work whenever I updated myself on octreotide research.

It seems that Prof Di Bella became convinced not only that he had discovered a new and effective approach to cancer treatment but also that this approach was so manifestly effective that it did not need to be subjected to the usual, and time-consuming, processes of sceptical enquiry, the null hypothesis and RCTs. His claim that it was good not just for selected cancers but for almost all varieties should been a warning sign. At some stage, he presumably communicated his evident enthusiasm to desperate patients and their equally desperate friends and relations and eventually, the Italian media got to hear about him. The words that Italians use for 'breakthrough', 'cure' and – no doubt – 'miracle' duly appeared in Italian newspapers and a 'movement' was formed. Unlike that earlier and more sinister Italian movement the *Movimento Soziale Italiano,* better known as the Fascists, they did not march *on* Rome, like Mussolini and his Blackshirts in 1922 but they certainly marched *in* the Eternal City and demonstrated outside the offices of the unfortunate Minister of Health. In December 1997, a judge, evidently influenced by media reports, ruled that the Italian health service, cash-strapped like most health services, should fund the treatment for a 2-year-old child with brain cancer. Several similar rulings followed. Italian pharmacies began to run out of octreotide. Six months later, the child died of his cancer.

It is perhaps slightly stretching the term to call the demonstrators 'ideological' but only slightly. Many of them had been diagnosed with cancers and were understandably desperate. Desperation itself is hardly an ideology, though when it comes to truth-claims, its effects can be just as undesirable and distorting as fervent nationalism, religious orthodoxy or an *a priori* conviction of the effectiveness of homoeopathy, acupuncture or psychoanalysis. However, there seem to have been some underlying beliefs that came close to ideology, such as that Prof Di Bella was a genius, that he had discovered a genuinely effective treatment and (a typical conspiracy theory) that his medical colleagues and the State were wilfully suppressing his discoveries for deplorable personal or economic reasons like pride, cost to the health service, competition and so forth. There was also an element of nationalism, since an Italian doctor had supposedly succeeded where other nations had failed. An Italian cancer specialist, Giovanni Bertelli, reported that: "Magazines, newspapers, and television stations — especially those linked to right-wing opposition parties — expressed support."[206]

If the Health Minister groaned when he heard the demonstrators outside his window, we must sympathise with him, for "When requested by the ministry of health to submit scientific evidence of the effectiveness of Di Bella multitherapy, Dr Di Bella failed to produce any published scientific paper".[207] Such was the pressure from the *Bellatisti* that instead of demanding, quite reasonably, that the professor should take his place in the queue of well-intentioned cancer researchers and do some clinical trials or animal studies, the Italian government felt obliged to set up a research group for the specific purpose of doing what the null hypothesis required that Di Bella himself ought to have done before making his claims. To reduce the risk that if the result were negative or unconvincing, Di Bella would simply criticize the design of the study, they invited him to join the planning group, as Prof Ernst did with spiritual healers in his own study. It is a testament to Di Bella's sincerity and conviction that he did so, though Bertelli reports: "Di Bella ... expressed fears that the results would be 'sabotaged' by mainstream doctors. He also accused drug companies of conspiring against him and even claimed he had been the target of an assassination attempt. The drama increased when Di Bella, speaking to European Parliament members, announced that his regimen is also effective against retinitis pigmentosa, multiple sclerosis, amyotrophic lateral sclerosis [a.k.a. motor neurone disease] and Alzheimer's disease, all of which have no known medical cure." As with claims of near-universal efficacy for homoeopathy, acupuncture and – at least for 'neurotic' illnesses – psychoanalysis, this ought to have sounded several warning bells. So should the discovery that:

> "[although] Di Bella had boasted that his personal files contained proof that he had cured thousands of patients ... his credibility was shaken by an analysis of 3076 of his records. According to the National Institute of Health, 1,553 (50%) contained no documentation that the patient had cancer, or lacked other essential information. Of the rest, 918 were excluded from further consideration because they lived in areas where tumor registries were not available, which meant that reliable survival information was not available either. Out of 605 patients living in areas covered by local tumor registries, only 248 had sufficient documentation of diagnosis and treatments. However, 244 of them had also received conventional treatments, which meant that no favorable conclusion could be drawn."

The study, nevertheless went ahead and its objective was quite modest – simply "To determine whether the treatment known as Di Bella multitherapy exerts antitumour activity worthy of further controlled clinical evaluation." In other words, the results only had to be promising or even encouraging, rather than conclusive. It would have been unethical to compare an unproved treatment with conventional, evidence-based ones and blinding would have been almost impossible but they did the next best thing. Since Di Bella treatment was demanded most loudly by people with cancers that had not responded to conventional treatment, they recruited "386 patients with advanced cancer...between March and July 1998 and followed to 31st October 1998." Some of them continued to have conventional treatment but most did not. They received every day "Melatonin, bromocriptine, either somatostatin or octreotide, and retinoid solution, the drugs that constitute Di Bella multitherapy." Although the study covered "eight different types of cancer [in] 26 Italian hospitals specialising in cancer treatment", the results should have put an end to the 'movement' and seem largely to have done so. DBM was, after all, "a multidrug, custom made medical treatment developed by Di Bella...who over the past 25 years has perfected and administered it on a private outpatient basis, claiming its effectiveness in blocking, if not curing altogether, most cancers." Yet of this fairly typical collection of Italians with advanced cancer, "No patient showed complete remission. Three patients showed partial remission: one of the 32 patients with non-Hodgkin's lymphoma;

one of the 33 patients with breast cancer; and one of the 29 patients with pancreatic cancer. At the second examination, 12% (47) of the patients had stable disease; 52% (199) progressed; and 25% (97) died." In other words, pretty much what would be expected with conventional treatment: and not one single 'cure'. Furthermore, despite claims that the treatment "supposedly had no toxic effects ... [a]dverse effects (nausea, vomiting, diarrhoea, neurological signs) were reported in 23% of patients, and 3.3% had to stop because of adverse effects." Bertelli concludes: "As with other unorthodox cancer treatments, the controversy over Di Bella's therapy caused unnecessary suffering for patients and their families. Media fervour, judicial decisions, and public pressure compelled the government to sponsor clinical trials despite the lack of scientific evidence. Predictably, results were negative. The trials helped calm public hysteria and kept some cancer patients from abandoning effective treatments. This was achieved, however, with considerable waste of precious government resources." Di Bella's son, also a physician, still carries a torch for his father's ideology but family loyalty is a notorious source of bias and worse.

Is it significant that the evidence-free doctrines of homoeopathy, discussed in the next chapter, are most strongly defended and propagated[208] in Germany, the nation of its founder? Nationalist bias and distortions in countries like Italy and Germany with a free press and democratic governments are even more likely to occur in totalitarian states like China and Cuba with neither. There are five times more papers about acupuncture on the PubMed website than about homoeopathy but less than a quarter of the 45,000 titles or abstracts mention controlled trials and not all of that quarter actually describe a controlled trial. That still leaves quite a lot of trials but where RCTs are concerned, quantity is no substitute for quality. The Cochrane Collaboration, brainchild of a British physician called Archie Cochrane who developed some of his ideas when he was the medical officer in a Nazi Prisoner of War camp, sets the pattern and standard for distinguishing good research from the mediocre, the bad and the frankly hopeless or corrupt. There are more examples in the last three categories than you might think and the quality of research in CAM is particularly poor. No country is free from badly-designed or actually fraudulent trials and the growth of 'vanity journals' that will publish almost anything, provided that authors or university departments pay them, has worsened the problem. However, national pride and cultural tradition can have distorting effects and they seem to be influential in Chinese research, especially, if unsurprisingly, where it involves acupuncture. An important scientific review of this problem was tellingly entitled: 'Do certain countries produce only positive results?[209] A *Lancet* editorial noted that: "fabrication, falsification, plagiarism, and unattributed ghost-writing threaten to overshadow China's achievements" and that "misconduct might not be limited to isolated individuals or institutions, but...could have infiltrated the country's research culture more widely".[210]

Cochrane Systematic Reviews of research evidence try very hard to be objective, transparent and unbiased. They use all relevant data – both published and, where obtainable, unpublished – and may use sophisticated statistical methods like meta-analysis in an attempt to provide the most robust estimates of treatment effects. The criteria for classifying RCTs by quality are openly stated and the data are available for anyone to check and criticize. Repeatedly, where acupuncture is the topic under review, their conclusion is that acupuncture has no specific effects or has only marginal and doubtful effects on minor symptoms, especially symptoms that are heavily influenced by psychological factors (including placebo effects) such as pain. Another regular conclusion is that there is simply insufficient high-quality evidence to permit a conclusion either way. As to those crucial 'meridians' and 'acupuncture points', even a meta-analysis published by the presumably CAM-friendly 'Division for Research and Education in Complementary and Integrative Medical Therapies' at Harvard concluded: "The studies were generally poor in quality... Based on this review, the evidence does not conclusively support the claim that acupuncture points or meridians are electrically distinguishable".[211]

The similarity between belief in undetectable but doctrinally crucial meridians and belief in undetectable but doctrinally crucial changes to consecrated bread and wine is not the only unfortunate feature of acupuncture research, most of which is done and published in China. If Italy's culture of corruption is an added reason for scepticism about the miracles validated by the Vatican's *Consulta Medica*, (see Ch 11) China, as of 2024, is even more corrupt at 76th out of 168 countries in Transparency International's Index and dropped three points from the previous year. The Chinese government itself admits that corruption is a serious problem but its Maoist history and current nationalist-autocratic political atmosphere are additional potential sources of academic bias. The only examples of real political, governmental censorship in conventional medicine that I know of involved doctors working in the health services of totalitarian communist countries such as present-day

Cuba and pre-1989 Russia. Doctors were reluctant to criticize locally developed theories or treatments because that could be very bad for their careers. Russian psychiatrists who questioned the existence of 'reformist delusions' and 'sluggish schizophrenia' (the uniquely Soviet mental illnesses that supposedly afflicted Russian dissidents) were themselves compulsorily detained in psychiatric hospitals. In Cuba, a country that I know and like and that has a rather good health service, two treatments developed there were claimed to be effective for retinitis pigmentosa (a hereditary and progressive form of blindness) and vitiligo, a less serious but often disfiguring skin disease. The former involved mixing the patient's blood with ozone and returning it to the circulation, or giving a kind of ozone enema. The latter involved an extract made from human placentas, easily available in one of the very few Latin American countries with woman-friendly abortion laws.

Neither of the treatments had been subjected to even a simple RCT in Cuba and nobody outside Cuba thought they were effective. A US before-and-after study of patients who had gone to Cuba for the ozone treatment was unable to show any benefit and even suggested that "this intervention may worsen the course of the disease".[212] One former Cuban doctor told me that he had risked escaping by boat to Florida because he became fed up with demands to falsify official health statistics. In the capitalist west, especially in the USA, we are brought up on the principle that if you build a better mousetrap, the world will beat a path to your door. In totalitarian countries, if you build a better mousetrap, the people who beat a path to your door, typically at 5am, may be the thought police asking why you aren't satisfied with the standard, official mousetrap, comrade. In such an atmosphere, randomised controlled trials and the null hypothesis may be very unwelcome if they contradict the party line. Lysenko's ghost is still active.[213] When nationalism combines with ideology and institutionalized corruption, it needs a lot of courage to ask embarrassing clinical questions that conflict with therapeutic jingoism and pose a serious risk to your career, happiness, income or even liberty. The monotheisms also tend to give short shrift to serious questioners.

It seems fitting to end with a very high-profile cases involving a man who was not only convinced that modern medicine didn't have all the answers (a conviction shared by all modern doctors) but also had a parallel belief that an alternative – or rather Alternative – treatment would be preferable, when he developed pancreatic cancer in his fifties. Cancer of the pancreas generally has a very poor prognosis, death usually occurring within a year or two with typical five-year survival rates of less than 20% for the commonest variety, adenocarcinoma. It has often spread and become inoperable by the time it is diagnosed and it does not respond well to conventional chemotherapy and radiotherapy. As it happened, Steve Jobs – the charismatic, idiosyncratic and very rich founder of Apple – developed a different and uncommon pancreatic cancer, an islet cell tumour, which is generally less malignant and has a reasonably encouraging prognosis with 5-year survival rates around 50%. Being rich meant that he could afford to doctor-shop. Being idiosyncratic seems to have meant that he was naturally attracted to idiosyncratic and CAM treatments. Rejecting advice to have conventional treatment, he opted for various diets recommended by CAM practitioners. By the time the relentless progression of the cancer persuaded him to change his mind, it was too late.[214] Jobs's death at 56 could probably have been postponed and might have been avoided. His ideological embrace of the unorthodox and counter-intuitive in medicine may not have been particularly fervent. It helped to make him very successful in the world of electronics but it was a poor basis for selecting medical treatment.

At least poor Steve Jobs's misplaced herbal and Alternative ideology prematurely ended only his own life. Similar ideological distortions inflicted on HIV-infected South Africans by ex-President Thabo Mbeki of South Africa and his health minister Dr. Manto Tshabalala-Msimang, a Soviet medical graduate, ensured that many tens of thousands died of AIDS in South Africa who could have been kept alive and in good health by the orthodox medical treatment that both politicians openly derided. The health minister notoriously advised HIV patients to rely on beetroot, lemon and garlic instead of anti-viral drugs. Even after leaving office, she was reported as saying that Africa should 'benefit more from its ancient traditional knowledge', without specifying which particular bits of beneficial 'traditional knowledge' she had in mind. It seems that combinations of nationalist and anti-scientific ideologies can sometimes cause even more deaths than plain, unaided nationalism.

Chapter 15
Homoeopathy: sweet nothings
The missing molecule mystery

Considering that enthusiasm moves the world, it is a pity that so few enthusiasts can be trusted to tell the truth.

Arthur Balfour, British Prime Minister, 1902-5

In the West, the oldest of the 'scripture-based' varieties of Complementary and Alternative Medicine is homoeopathy. It is also the only one that has had a politically significant foothold in the NHS, though never a clinically significant one, modern homoeopaths being noticeably reluctant to treat life-threatening illnesses with their nostrums. Most modern critics of homoeopathy focus, quite reasonably, on the RCTs that have shown its treatments and at least some of its practitioners to have useful placebo effects but nothing more. In this chapter my focus will mainly be on the arrogance and grandiosity of its guru-like originator because these characteristics should have made people doubt his claims long before the RCTs demolished them.

Just as one man, Sigmund Freud, was the father of psychoanalysis, Samuel Hahnemann was the founding father of homoeopathy. If I devote less space here to Hahnemann's personality than to Freud's later in the book, that is only because we know less about him than we do about Freud, though we know more than enough. These remarks are not a prelude to general *ad hominem* criticisms because in this context, I really don't care whether or not Hahnemann and Freud were cruel to animals, unfaithful to their wives, revolting in their personal habits or malevolent in their social and political views. What I do care about – and what I think it is quite reasonable to bring up in any discussion of the history of a particular treatment – are any signs that the founders of homoeopathy and psychoanalysis realised how easy it is to mislead themselves and others about the true effectiveness of treatment. Did they know about placebo and non-specific effects, the natural history of diseases, regression to the mean or the null hypothesis? Did they understand the dangers of enthusiasm, self-deception and dogmatism? Were they in the habit of making unjustified claims about the real usefulness of their inventions? As a later chapter documents, most of these snares and delusions were obvious to the King of England and doubtless to other thoughtful people by the early 1600s.

Most of the following examples of Hahnemann's views are drawn from a translation[215] of the sixth and final 1842 edition of his *Organon of Medicine*. The translators themselves begin on a note of dogmatic euphoria. The book "clearly and completely states, for the first time in history, the *true nature of health and disease*.[my emphasis] ... It has remained until today the one essential cornerstone of homoeopathy, the ultimate authority on its doctrine and practice". The second claim may well be true. The first cannot possibly be. Hahnemann (whose final years of a long life were apparently blighted by asthma that was evidently unresponsive to homoeopathy) could not possibly have understood the 'true nature of health and disease' because he was born well before most of the important discoveries about the physiology and microscopic structure of our organs and of the bacterial and viral infections and other processes that damage or destroy them. Hahnemann, like all ideologists, had several Big Ideas, to which he adhered as a matter of fundamental – not to say fundamentalist – principle. The Big Ideas were even more important to him than to some other ideologues because while Lenin and Stalin were devoted and convinced Marxists, they did not claim to have invented Marxism or Communism. Hahnemann, in contrast, not only thought that the Big Ideas of homoeopathy were true: he also claimed to have been their sole inventor. This naturally increased his personal, emotional investment in the Ideas and surely made it even more difficult than usual to accept even the possibility that he might have been wrong.

Let me, though, readily acknowledge that one thing Hahnemann got right about the conventional medical treatments of his era – even if he was right without having any really convincing evidence at the time – was that many of them were not only without specific effectiveness but also actively harmful, as we have already discussed. Blood-letting, in particular, was enthusiastically practised by doctors and requested by patients. Only in the late 19th century did the increasing understanding of blood and the circulation show that for most conditions, blood-letting was likely to impede recovery and could be lethal (as it probably was for George Washington). The only things for which it is still indicated are a small group of rather rare diseases, some of them unknown until the last half-century, in which there is an excess of certain blood cells, or of iron. Hahnemann could not have known it in any objective, scientific way but he felt – either instinctively or from uncontrolled observation, or both – that blood-letting was harmful. He did not, as far as we know, work it out from experiment or from an accurate understanding of the physiology of blood and circulation. He could therefore just as easily have been wrong and was lucky rather than particularly clever; or, if you prefer it, he was right for the wrong reasons.

Hahnemann's first Big Idea was that apart from injuries, all illnesses – and he really meant *all* – were caused by disturbances in the 'Vital Force'. He never clearly defines this Force (the idea of 'vitalism' was common at the time) but merely makes the simple analogy that invisible forces - invisible, that is, to the unaided eyes of the 18th and early 19th centuries - are involved in gravity and magnetism. They must therefore be involved in health and disease as well, QED.

> "As far as the physician is concerned, is not that which reveals itself to the senses in symptoms the very disease itself? He can never see the immaterial element, the vital force causing the disease. He need never see it; to cure he needs only to see and understand its morbific [i.e. disease-causing] effects. ... So it is the totality of symptoms, *the outer image expressing the inner essence of the disease, i.e. of the disturbed vital force* that must be the main, even the only means by which the disease allows us to find the necessary remedy " (italics original p. 12)

The next Big Idea soon follows.

> "Outer malefic agents that harm the healthy organism and disturb the harmonious rhythm of life can reach and affect the spirit-like *dynamis* only in a way that also is dynamic and spirit-like. The physician can remove these pathological untunements (diseases) only by acting on our spirit-like vital force with medicines having equally spirit-like dynamic effects that are perceived by the nervous sensitivity everywhere present in the organism. So it is only by dynamic action on the vital principle that remedies can restore health and the harmony of life..." (p. 21 Italics original)

So, this mysterious, invisible, un-measurable, all-permeating and in every sense 'vital' force (for "without the vital force, the body dies" (p. 15) is present not only in living bodies but in all substances, including most particularly those substances, even minerals, administered in the hope of relieving disease. Mysterious, invisible, un-measurable, all-permeating: it's already beginning to sound very like the traditional attributes of the monotheistic or trinitarian god. Hahnemann insisted that in order to maximise, or 'potentise', the invisible and un-measurable vital force in the medicines he proposed to use, they had to be prepared in a particular way.

> "By [this] special procedure, never tried before my time, homoeopathy develops the inner, spirit-like medicinal powers of substances to a degree hitherto unheard of and makes all of them exceedingly, even immeasurably, penetrating, active and effective ... This remarkable transformation develops the latent *dynamic* powers previously imperceptible [that] electively affect the vital principle of animal life". (p. 188 Italics original)

I will return to this 'special procedure' shortly.

"Never tried before my time". Variations on this refrain appear very frequently in Hahnemann's writing. Indeed, few medical writers illustrate so perfectly Sir Francis Bacon's observation four centuries ago that; "men fall in love with particular pieces of knowledge and thoughts; either because they believe themselves to be their authors and inventors; or because they have put a great deal of labour into them and have got very used to them".

Here are a few examples of Hahnemann's Hubris:

"I was the first to tread this path. And my steadfastness of purpose came about and was sustained only because I was completely convinced of the great truth and blessing to mankind that the homoeopathic use of medicines was the only certain way in which it was possible to cure human diseases". [p. 99-100, my italics]

"It took me twelve years of research to find the source of this incredible number of chronic diseases, to investigate and confirm this great truth hidden from all my predecessors and contemporaries and to discover the ... remedies that are usually able to deal with this thousand-headed monster in its widely varying forms and manifestations". [p. 78-9, my italics]

What was this hydra-like 'source' of so much human misery? The cause of "neurasthenia, hysteria, hypochondria, mania, melancholia, idiocy, madness, epilepsy and all kinds of fits, softening of the bones (rachitis) [rickets], scrofula, scoliosis and kyphosis, bone caries, cancer, fungus haematodes, neoplasms, gout, haemorrhoids, jaundice and cyanosis, dropsy, amenorrhoea, haemorrhage of the stomach, nose, lungs, bladder and womb, asthma and suppuration of the lungs, impotence and infertility, migraine, deafness, cataract and amaurosis [blindness], kidney stones, paralyses, deficiencies of the senses, and every kind of pain etc, all mentioned in pathology books as separate diseases"? (p 78) Well, it is something called 'psora'. The word means 'itch' in Greek (the skin disease psoriasis doesn't usually itch, though it may do) and at one time it seems to have been particularly used to describe scabies (which certainly does itch). However, when one tries to find out what the word means to homoeopaths, it turns out to be very ill-defined. It isn't explained in the *Organon* and a search of homoeopathic websites gives several interpretations. Here is an example from the website of an Indian homoeopath. "Had psora never been established as a miasm upon the human race, the other two chronic diseases would have been impossible, and susceptibility to acute diseases would have been impossible. All the diseases of man are built upon psora ; hence it is the foundation of sickness; all other sickness came afterwards. Psora is the underlying cause, and is the primitive or primary disorder of the human race. It is a disordered state of the internal economy of the human race. This state expresses itself in the forms of the varying chronic diseases, or chronic manifestations. If the human race had remained in a state of perfect order, psora could not have existed. The susceptibility to psora opens out a question altogether too broad to study among the sciences in a medical College. It is altogether too extensive, for it goes to the very primitive wrong of the human race, the very first sickness of the human race, that is the spiritual sickness, from which first state the race progressed into what may be called the true susceptibility to psora, which in turn laid the foundation for other diseases."[216] *'If the human race had remained in a state of perfect order, psora could not have existed.'* Doesn't that sound very like the myth of the Garden of Eden – a pre-lapsarian world free of pain, disease and sin?

Here are two more definitions. "The itching is the manifestation of Psora. Psora being the condition of a system enabling it to develop disease. Psora in itself is invisible, it is the effects of Psora that are visible and are also innumerable. The very basis of disease from which all eruptive diseases of the Earth originated is Psoric."[217] "The word miasm means a cloud or fog in the being. The theory suggests that if 100% of all disease is miasmatic, then 85% is due to the primary and atavistic miasm Hahnemann called Psora. The remaining 15% of all disease he held to be either syphilitic or sycotic,[sic – it means 'relating to the skin' and is not a mis-spelling of 'psychotic'] being derived from suppressed Syphilis or suppressed Gonorrhoea."[218] As well as their unhelpful and quasi-theological vagueness, these extracts demonstrate the all-embracing, universal claims of homoeopathy that are also typical of much religious discourse.

As impressive and comprehensive as the list of conditions caused by psora are the repeated and confident assertions in *Organon* that homoeopathy can "almost without exception bring about perfect cures":

> (p.79) "There could not possibly be any true, best way of curing dynamic (i.e. all non-surgical) diseases other than pure homoeopathy, just as one could not possibly draw more than one straight line between two given points" (p.100); "there are but few cases of disease left for which a relatively suitable homoeopathic remedy cannot be found from among the medicines so far proved. *Such a remedy restores health easily, surely, mildly and permanently*". [p.120. my italics]

Big Idea number three – probably the best-known homoeopathic notion – did not follow naturally from the previous two, though it had no more evidence to support it than they did. This was the idea that 'like cures like' – that symptoms of particular illnesses can be cured by small doses of drugs which, in 'normal' doses, can produce, as desired effects or as side effects, those very same symptoms. Rendered into Latin as *'similia similibus curentur'*, it has the same impressive, comforting ring that fine old Latin phrases can have in other contexts (especially religious ones like the Latin Tridentine Mass) or that political slogans have in revolutionary circles. I have long had a theory about the eureka moment that apparently caused Hahnemann to conceive this crucial pillar of homoeopathic treatment. As is well documented, Hahnemann took an extract of cinchona bark (also called 'fever bark' or 'Peruvian bark') as an experiment and became briefly feverish afterwards. We know now that the therapeutically active ingredient of cinchona bark is quinine but Hahnemann couldn't have known that at the time, since quinine wasn't isolated until 1818. As is pretty obvious, quinine does not usually cause fevers, otherwise many of us would feel feverish after a gin and tonic. It can, however, cause reversible tinnitus, which has happened to people after drinking too much tonic water, and even blindness.[219]

It is possible, of course, that in Hahnemann's case, the fever and the administration of quinine were coincidental rather than causally related; and that the crucial conclusion that he drew from his initial observation was thus erroneous from the start, though he apparently repeated the experiment more than once with similar results. However, an alternative explanation is that Hahnemann had some sort of allergy or hypersensitivity to quinine, or perhaps to some other constituent of cinchona bark. (A problem with all herbal medicines is that you never know which of the many compounds in a plant extract is the crucial and supposedly therapeutic one.) Hahnemann might have had a common and genetically determined deficiency of the enzyme glucose-6-phosphate dehydrogenase (G6PD), a deficiency known to be associated with toxic reactions, including feverish ones, to several common drugs, including quinine, and also to certain foods, notably broad beans. I cannot find a mention of this possible explanation in PubMed but an undated internet article by Dr W E Thomas[220] makes the same suggestion. Whichever explanation is correct, Hahnemann's mistaken conclusion that quinine can cause fever in healthy people (mistaken because quinine doesn't normally cause fever and because people with G6PD deficiency are, by definition, not physiologically and biochemically normal and may become unhealthy because of their abnormality) led him to construct a whole 'grand theory' to which everything subsequently had to become subservient, as happened with Christianity, Islam and Communism. The 'holy books' could not be fundamentally questioned without loss of face and loss of authority.

Imbued with the ideas that 'like cures like' and that the 'vital spirit' of both patients and medicines had to be fostered and strengthened, Hahnemann's next Big Idea was even more imaginative. Where medicines were concerned, he proclaimed *ex cathedra* that less was more. The higher the dilution and thus the lower the dose, the more therapeutically potent a particular remedy would allegedly be. The idea was that the water in which these increasingly scarce molecules were diluted retained, in some mysterious way, a 'memory' of the molecule that was – in some other and equally mysterious way – therapeutic. Homoeopaths maintain that this mysterious power exists even though nobody (including homoeopaths) has been able to demonstrate it.

These claims are very like those made for the Blessed Sacrament or Eucharist that plays such a central role in the service of Holy Communion in the Roman Catholic church. Worried that many of his flock misunderstood the nature of transubstantiation, or doubted it altogether, Archbishop Michael Sheehan of Santa Fé in New Mexico tried to make it clear. The change in the nature of the sacramental bread and wine "happens during the eucharistic prayer of the Mass. At that time, the bread and wine are changed into the Body and Blood of Christ, as the Church has always taught. Although they still look like bread and wine, they have, by divine power, actually changed into His Body and Blood. How can we know this? It requires faith. It is a mystery which, like love, we will never fully understand."[221] This lack of understanding does not stop the Vatican from having firm views on what types of bread can and cannot be changed in this way and I'm afraid that gluten-free is out. "Hosts that are completely gluten-free are invalid matter for the celebration of the Eucharist."[222] "The Holy See has declared that some gluten is necessary for the substance to be considered as true bread. And thus a gluten-free wafer, in spite of its external resemblance, is no longer bread and thus is incapable of becoming the Body of Christ."[223] How, in God's name, can they possibly know that?

It was not enough for homoeopathic drugs to be progressively diluted well beyond the point at which a single molecule of the drug in question was likely to be found in the spoonful or pill given to the patient. Before dilution, the fluid extract also had to be 'succussed', which means it had to be hit against a soft leather pad exactly one hundred times (though at one stage, Hahnemann apparently thought that hitting it against a Bible would be even better.) One hundred is an example of a 'magic number', like 3 or 7 or 49 or 666. It was another of Hahnemann's *ex cathedra* statements and until very recently, this absolutely fundamental claim that succussion was vital to maximising the effectiveness of homoeopathic medicines had never been objectively tested. It still hasn't been subjected to the sort of concentrated attention and carefully controlled studies that it surely deserves, given its centrality to homoeopathic doctrine but recently, succussion was examined as part of a controlled study of the effect of various homoeopathic remedies on sleep.[224] As usual, it was published in a journal that is devoted almost entirely to homoeopathy, which means that right from the start, its credibility is reduced. If it was peer-reviewed, the peer-reviewers would almost certainly not have had the questioning, sceptical attitudes that are the essence of the scientific method. The study compared no succussion (stirred but not shaken, as it were) with 20, 40 and 100 succussions. There were indeed some slight differences between the succussion groups but they were not in any consistent direction. In other words, there was no evidence in what seems to be first study to address the issue, even though it wasn't its main focus, that more succussion had bigger effects than less, as claimed, very insistently, by Hahnemann and his past and present disciples. One homoeopathy supporter even assured a House of Commons committee that mere stirring wouldn't do the job.[225] As Guy Chapman, an engineer by profession, has commented: "Let's not forget that in order for homeopathy to be right, everything we know about the nature of matter, human biochemistry, pharmacology, aetiology [causation] and numerous other fields must be not just wrong but spectacularly wrong."[226]

I wonder, incidentally, how a quality-control inspector could possibly confirm the composition of a remedy claiming to have a 'potency' of 50x (i.e. serially diluted 50 times) when it is rather unlikely that the bottle would contain even a single molecule of the substance in question? How, come to that, could the inspector determine whether the medicine had really been 'succussed' (i.e. ritually shaken) one hundred times, as required by homoeopathic theory, rather than some cheapskate version succussed only ten times or not succussed at all?

The fact is, there is no scientific test known to man (or woman) that can distinguish between a sample of a homoeopathic remedy and a sample of pure distilled water.

In Hahnemann's time, most medicines were herbal and homoeopathy naturally reflects that part of its history. Some herbalist doctrines and therefore some homoeopathic ones reflect other varieties of 'magical thinking'. During the 1970s, one of Queen Elizabeth's physicians at Buckingham Palace was a homoeopathic doctor (i.e. a qualified doctor who mainly used homoeopathy) called Dr Margery Blackie and she had written a book about homoeopathy that was sent to me for review.[227] The section of her book that made me instantly regard homoeopathy as a branch of witch-doctoring was her reason for recommending a homoeopathic preparation of pulsatilla in paediatrics:

> "[The] very changeable child may often go faint in a hot room…They are thirstless children who hate fat and like sweet things…and at night will sleep with their arms above their heads. We treat these children with their fluctuating temperaments and physiques with Pulsatilla which comes from the *pulsatilla vulgaris* 'the wind flower' remedy [which] like the patient is very changeable, and is often referred to as the 'weathercock remedy'."

I'm not sure what she means by 'changeable' but in non-homoeopathic doses, pulsatilla can be extremely toxic to the heart. The pulsatilla entry on the 2016 website of the British Homoeopathic Association says nothing about "thirstless children who hate fat and like sweet things" and now claims that "Pulsatilla is predominantly a female remedy. It is classically thought to suit blonde, blue-eyed females of a mild, shy and tearful disposition."[228] Take your pick.

Thus, in the last quarter of the 20th century, one of the leaders of British homoeopathy propagated this sort of primitive, magical thinking, no different in principle from the magical thinking behind the votive offerings that the sick used to leave at shrines; small representations of a hand, a foot or a phallus, which it was hoped the presiding deity would restore to health. That homoeopathy ever occupied its small, shrinking and now barely visible enclave in the NHS probably owes something to royal patronage dating back to well before King Charles III was born. For although touching by Royalty for the 'King's Evil'[229] may have ended with the death of Queen Anne in 1714, the adulation and emulation of all things Royal have not.[230] Soon after moving into Buckingham Palace King Charles appointed a CAM- and homoeopathy-friendly GP, Dr Michael Dixon, as the head of the Royal Medical Household. After reading an interview he gave to *The Times* in 2024, I rather warm to the man but his views on homoeopathy are so atypical of homoeopaths and so important in their implications that he merits several paragraphs in the Conclusion.

As well as sympathetic magic, the 'wind flower' claim is a variant of another ancient idea, the 'Doctrine of Signatures', which is probably at least as old as Hippocrates. It embodies the magical idea that plants with an appearance suggestive of a particular organ should be useful in treating disorders of that organ. Thus, the leaves of lungwort, which have a spotted appearance vaguely (very vaguely) reminiscent of the surface of lungs, were used for treating supposed lung disorders, even though breathing difficulties are often primarily due to heart disease rather than lung disease. Bloodroot, popular for presumed 'disorders of the blood', produces a blood-red juice. It is very poisonous and could certainly have caused some impressive toxic effects that might have persuaded patients that it was a powerful remedy, if they survived, on the principle that good medicines taste nasty. Liverwort leaves have the shape of livers. You get the idea.

Early in the 17th century, the Protestant mystic Jakob Boehme promoted an addition to the Doctrine of Signatures; the doctrine that God had provided these 'signatures' for our benefit. This was doubtless an attractive add-on when religion was so central to everyday life in Europe, though Boehme died, probably of cancer, aged only 49. There are herbalists and other CAM practitioners today who encourage their patients to take useless or poisonous plant medicines in place of well-researched treatments that might actually save their lives, but it is not only humans who suffer from these seductive absurdities. The same primitive, magical thinking has led to the near-extermination of the blameless rhinoceros just because its horn has a suggestive shape and is therefore supposed to make men horny, among other alleged properties. O libido: what crimes are committed in thy name! Such superstitions are bad for reason and rhinos alike. A more animal-friendly variant of this process of magical thinking and 'signatures' was the belief that particular saints had the ability to heal particular parts of the body, though in this case, the matching of disease or organ to saint was based not on the saint's physical appearance or historical associations but on the saint's name. "Saint Pissoux was supposed to be good for urinary infections, Saint Bavard [bavarder means to chat or gossip] for mutes and Saint Clair ('clear') for the short-sighted ... In Normandy, reciting the service of the Toussaint (All Saints Day) was thought to be good for people with a cold because Toussaint sounds like *tousser* (to cough)."[231]

Plant-based drugs are incorporated into scientific medicine when they are supported by RCTs and there are surely more to come but as with 'traditional Chinese medicine', the fact that infant mortality was so high and that many adults died of acute illnesses before they reached even 50 suggests that this ancient Occidental wisdom was not very useful to them. Herbal enthusiasts often imply that anything 'natural' is basically Good, while nasty, synthetic drugs are basically Bad, but adverse effects do not respect ideologies. I first saw the damage that 'natural' herbs could cause when I worked in Jamaica in 1970. Black Jamaicans were then prone to a type of cirrhosis of the liver that was rarely seen in other countries or in other Jamaicans. It turned out to be due to a traditional 'natural' medicine known as 'bush tea', popular among Black Jamaicans, though not among Jamaica's other ethnic groups, as a cure-all or general pick-me-up and often given to children as well as adults. This life-threatening cirrhosis was apparently due to a component from one particular plant, a local variety of *vinca* or periwinkle. The *vinca* genus contains, among other compounds, an alkaloid so toxic that in small and carefully measured doses, it has been used to suppress the bone marrow of patients with certain types of leukaemia. However, it was the sinister, white-coated scientists (some of them doubtless compounding their sinisterness by experimenting on cuddly, anthropomorphic creatures) and not the colourful Jamaican peasants in touch with Earth Wisdom, who discovered this single, genuinely therapeutic effect of *vinca* alkaloids, undreamed of by the mothers who fed poisonous bush tea to their offspring, or by the 'Obeah Men' (the local witch-doctors) who presumably recommended it. As a cause of cirrhosis in Jamaica, bush tea was exceeded at the time only by alcohol. Among its younger victims was a one-year old child.[232] However, a taste for hepatotoxic (i.e. liver-damaging) herbs is not restricted to the less sophisticated inhabitants of Jamaica. Noting that "Use of herbal and dietary supplements accounts for an increasing proportion of drug hepatotoxicity cases" a large US survey found that "an estimated 15.6 million US adults consumed at least one botanical product with [hepatotoxic] liability within the past 30 days, comparable with the number of people who consumed nonsteroidal anti-inflammatory drugs ... Clinicians should be aware of possible adverse events from consumption of these largely unregulated products".[233] The commonest supplements were 'turmeric or curcumin, green tea extract, Garcinia cambogia, black cohosh, red yeast rice, and ashwagandha". My local pharmacist told me that about 25% of his income comes from sales of dietary supplements and vitamins that in most cases will bring absolutely no specific biological benefit to those who consume them. A 2024 US study found no difference in mortality between consumers and non-consumers of multivitamins[234] but a diet containing olive oil, as is universal in southern Europe, may reduce dementia risk.[235] As with the gold-plated placebo pills, the more expensive the supplements and vitamins, the greater the degree of therapeutic delusion motivating their purchase.

Because China is a very large country, it is home to many indigenous plants and every now and then, a new one is discovered or an old one turns out to have some genuinely useful properties. Just as quinine-containing 'fever bark' proved to be a useful treatment for malaria, so did *artemisia annui,* a member of the wormwood family. The active chemical, artemisinin, was a useful addition to the existing range of antimalarials but resistant strains of the malaria parasite are now established. It is also more efficiently produced by synthesis than by harvesting. Might its Nobel-prize winning discovery have given Chinese herbal medicines an undeserved boost that most traditional Chinese herbs probably do not merit?

Sometimes, herbal remedies were praised and recommended for effects that were not merely imaginary but the opposite of their real pharmacological mechanisms. Nicholas Culpepper's 'Complete Herbal and English Physician', the standard 17th C textbook and still in print, was enthusiastic about willow bark to "stanch bleeding of wounds ... spitting of blood and other fluxes of blood in man or woman".[236] In reality, the bark of the willow tree (*salix*) contains salicylic acid, the basis of aspirin which, far from stanching bleeding, is a powerful anti-clotting agent, taken by millions of people today for that very purpose as well as for its rather modest pain-relieving and anti-inflammatory properties.

When pre-scientific medicines had a rapid effect, or when they were used to treat easily visible organs, our therapeutic forebears might sometimes strike lucky. Thus, whoever chewed the first opium poppy-head or made the first poppy-tea infusion would have soon experienced the tranquillising, dream-inducing, analgesic and diarrhoea-relieving effects of crude opium, which typically contains 10-20% of morphine. Provided, that is, he didn't overdo it, since there may be enough morphine in a single poppy head to cause dangerous respiratory depression, especially in small children. Similarly, the Andean Amerindians who first chewed coca leaves, like their East African counterparts who chewed khat leaves, would soon have noticed their stimulating, energising effects. The same goes for the effects of the alcohol in naturally fermented fruit juices.

None of this criticism will go down well with the many people (and many patients) who feel that as with acupuncture and religion, those old beliefs must have *something* in them, even if scientists say otherwise. Let Rudyard Kipling have the last word.

Our fathers of old.
Excellent herbs had our fathers of old
Excellent herbs to ease their pain...
...Anything green that grew of the mould
Was an excellent herb to our fathers of old.

Wonderful little, when all is said,
Wonderful little our fathers knew.
Half their remedies cured you dead -
Most of their teaching was quite untrue -
"Look at the stars when a patient is ill
(Dirt has nothing to do with disease.)
Bleed and blister as much as you will,
Blister and bleed him as oft you please".
Whence enormous and manifold
Errors were made by our fathers of old. [237]

Chapter 16
One-shot healers and one-shot priests
If your only tool is a hammer, all problems look like nails

Another shared characteristic of religion and CAM is that many practitioners know how to play only one therapeutic tune. There is some dispute about who first warned us that 'If your only tool is a hammer, all your problems start to look like nails' but nowhere is that more true than in organised religion and CAM.

During the past century, it has been rare for CAM techniques and their religious equivalents to be actively discarded on the grounds of total or relative ineffectiveness. New ones – mostly variations on the old ones – are usually just added to the pile of existing CAM treatments and existing religious sects, though some have faded away. In contrast, even the recent history of medicine is full of treatments that are no longer used. In some cases, despite early promise, they were found to be ineffective, or more harmful than beneficial, or simply harmful with no redeeming features at all. More often, especially in the last 40 years or so, it is because better treatments were developed, leaving the older ones to wither on the vine of progress. This sometimes meant that doctors who specialised in a particular treatment or a particular disease found themselves out of a job, because it could now be treated or prevented by GPs without involving hospitals or specialists, as happened with the treatment of gastric and duodenal ulcers. During my training, I often assisted at operations to treat ulcers that were causing pain but ulcers could also bleed profusely or ulcerate through the wall of the stomach or the duodenum. That required emergency intervention and was sometimes fatal. It still can be fatal, especially in the elderly but surgeons now see comparatively few ulcers because of a discovery in 1989 that showed that peptic ulcers were actually caused by a bacterium rather than stress or hyperacidity, leading to a simple method of prevention or treatment with cheap medicines that have so few serious side effects that they are sold without prescription in most countries.

The ulcer specialists had to use their surgical skills in some other field, retraining if necessary. The same happened with thoracic surgery for tuberculosis, which used to be common but virtually disappeared when effective anti-tuberculosis drugs were developed in the late 1940s. (George Orwell died in 1950 aged only 46 from advanced tuberculosis, just a few months too soon to benefit from one of the first RCTs, which showed streptomycin to be curative.)

The discovery that a widely-used or widely-recommended medical treatment actually has no specific effect or has unacceptable side-effects is rarer than it used to be because new treatments generally have to demonstrate their effectiveness and safety in controlled trials before they are widely adopted. Such discoveries pose no fundamental threat to the self-image, public image, income or employment of physicians or surgeons because there are many other effective treatments that they can use. Even if they have specialised exclusively in a subsequently-rejected treatment, they can brush up their old therapeutic and diagnostic skills or learn some new ones. They need never be without a medical job. More importantly, they do not have to defend the indefensible in order to maintain a reasonable income or to preserve their self-esteem. This is not the case with acupuncturists, homoeopaths, chiropractors and so forth, who often practice only one type of CAM and may thus have very powerful financial and emotional vested interests in maintaining the status of their particular corner of CAM and believing in its effectiveness. The blogger Guy Chapman puts this financial dilemma into comic relief. "In medicine, evidence must pass the test of *robustness*. In alternative-to-medicine [i.e. CAM] the test is *gobustness*: if I admit this result, will I go bust? If the answer is yes, then the evidence is considered refuted."

As it happens, during the last 30 years of my medical career, I tried hard to persuade largely sceptical or uninterested colleagues that two pharmacologically distinct drugs could be useful in the treatment of certain addictions. One of them used to be a routine treatment for alcoholism but had become unfashionable by the 1970s. Controlled studies from the 1970s onwards backed me up but I might have died without feeling really vindicated had I not lived long enough to see the publication of the three 'gold standard' Cochrane-style reviews that confirmed my views[238,239,240,241] I had a similar vindication with the other drug, used for heroin addiction,[242, 243, 244] but even if the research had shown that I was entirely wrong about both treatments and that they were actually no better than appropriate placebo controls, they constituted only a part of my practice and they thus completely failed the *'gobustness'* test. My academic reputation and self-esteem might have been badly dented but not my income, because there were several other more conventional and accepted addiction treatments that I also used. As a doctor with specialist psychiatric qualifications, I could also have returned to practising general psychiatry; or brushed up my knowledge of family planning, venereology or tropical diseases and made a late entry into an entirely different branch of medical practice.

Similar considerations apply in the case of the clergy, though in their case, disillusionment with a particular sect does not come from the results of controlled trials but from within. I have already discussed what happens to priests who lose their faith, especially if they lose it in mid-life or later and if they and their families live in houses that come (and go) with the job. The fact that most priests rely on a limited repertoire of interventions – prayer, pilgrimage, laying-on of hands, access to holy relics etc – does not, usually, worry their parishioners because they will generally share the priest's belief that these interventions are effective and appropriate. After all, both parties have usually been brought up to believe in them since early childhood. It does not usually worry the doctors of the sick parishioners either, because in the major Christian churches of the West, priests render unto the Caesar of medicine what belongs to Caesar and unto God what belongs to God. They do not commonly advise supplicants to abandon or reject orthodox medical interventions for diseases (as opposed to interventions for avoiding unwelcome pregnancy, in the case of Catholicism).

Exceptions to this co-existence are found mainly in some Pentecostal African and Afro-Caribbean churches that have advised HIV-infected parishioners to put their trust solely in God and throw away their truly life-saving medication. (It is called HAART – Highly Active Anti-Retroviral Therapy – because it really is Highly Active.) Some American churches, notably Christian Scientists, have the rejection of medicine at the heart of their ideology but Christian Science is one of the religions that is fading away. Reluctance or even refusal to co-exist is also common among CAM practitioners who quite often advise their patients to stop conventional medical treatments, even though this has resulted in well-documented cases of diseases like malaria that could have been prevented, cured or at least contained with evidence-based treatment. In some countries, Islamic preachers have issued *fatwas* against polio vaccination but this probably reflects a conspirationist belief that vaccination is part of a Western plot to sterilise Muslims, rather than a fundamental rejection of Western medicine.

Not all patients who consult homoeopaths or acupuncturists do so because they are already convinced that the underlying doctrines of causation and treatment are correct but many do. In the same way, many but not all of the pilgrims to Knock, Lourdes and Medjugorje are probably convinced that a timely offering or prayer can persuade God to reverse biological, mechanical and bacterial processes or to frustrate the wiles of Satan. As previously touched on, neither the already-convinced acupuncture patients nor the already-convinced Catholics would be likely to welcome the offer of even a small therapeutic menu containing chiropractic, crystal healing or Ayurvedic interventions, on the one hand, and Islamic or Buddhist holy relics on the other. However, apart from people who are committed to an 'alternative' lifestyle that is suspicious of all orthodoxies, patients may consult CAM practitioners in an opportunistic or tentative fashion, rather than from any firm *a priori* belief. Often, they do so after disappointing experiences with conventional medicine and may have no profound faith in any particular CAM treatment, let alone in CAM as a whole. There are still several conditions, particularly those with a large psychological component, for which conventional medicine does not have any satisfactory solutions and sometimes, the diagnosis itself may be far from certain. Nevertheless, if patients decide to make a start with – say – acupuncture, it is very unlikely that the acupuncturist they consult will immediately tell them that for their particular problem, homoeopathy or chiropractic would suit them better; or vice versa, though some CAM practitioners display a degree of therapeutic ecumenicalism that would get them admonished or de-frocked if they were Catholic priests. Since nearly all CAM procedures are placebos, at one level this does not matter much.

Chapter 17
The Katyn Massacre syndrome
'My enemy's enemy is my friend'

Let us re-recapitulate. Scientific, evidence-based medicine, like science in general, constantly reviews, criticises and re-evaluates its own practices and theories. When it has time and funds, it may do the same for the practices and theories of Complementary and Alternative Medicine if it can avoid the sort of obstacles that were placed in the way of Prof. Edzard Ernst at Exeter medical school by people not a million miles from the court of King Charles.[245] Proper scientists have to do this work because, unfortunately, the practitioners of CAM often don't get round either to doing it or even to recognising the need for doing it. Furthermore, research published by CAM practitioners in all countries tends to be low on quality and credibility, as judged by the criteria applied to orthodox medical research. However, I do not think that all or even most CAM practitioners are charlatans, i.e. doing and/or promoting *for essentially commercial reasons* something they know to be without specific effect. This surely means that among their number, there are practitioners with serious reservations about some of the mainstream treatments practised inside the very broad church of CAM, never mind the more marginal cults. There may even be CAM equivalents of the disillusioned priests mentioned earlier; practitioners in their 40s or 50s who have lost their faith in homoeopathy or acupuncture or CAM in general but could not easily make a comparable living in some other type of work.

It is rare for any of the CAM practitioners engaged in this kind of effectiveness research to voice fundamental criticism of particular CAM treatments, theories or practitioners. One likely reason is that by drawing attention to the lack of evidence for one particular underlying theory, there is a risk that the shortage of good evidence for other theories of CAM will be highlighted. Individual CAM practitioners may (and often do) have strong views about which CAM procedures are most appropriate for particular conditions but while they naturally tend to recommend their own favourite treatment ('If your only tool is a hammer...') they rarely criticise their competitors in public. CAM practitioners have enough sense to realise that, as Benjamin Franklin joked during the American War of Independence, if they don't hang together, they may hang separately.

In the 1990s, Dr Robert Park attended a press conference called by the predecessor of what is now the US National Institutes of Health's Office of Alternative Medicine. (The organisation was set up after pressure from, in particular, a US senator who claimed that he had been cured of his allergies by bee pollen. The senatorial pollen was supplied by a man who insisted, among other things, that "the risen Jesus Christ, when he came back to earth, consumed bee pollen".) "Perhaps the strangest part of the press conference." Park reported, "consisted of brief statements by individual members of the editorial review board of what they saw as the most important issues. ... One insisted that the number-one health problem in the United States is magnesium deficiency; another was convinced that the expanded use of acupuncture could revolutionise medicine and so it went around the table. ... There was no sense of conflict or rivalry. As each spoke, the other would nod in agreement. The purpose ... I began to realise, was to demonstrate that these disparate therapies all work. It was my first glimpse of what it is that holds alternative medicine together: there is no internal dissent in a community that feels itself besieged from the outside."[246] Barker Bausell, who cites the report in *Snake Oil Science*, says that he observed this type of behaviour "numerous times during [his] own involvement" in an NIH-funded centre for CAM research.

In recent years, we have seen a religious version of this sort of coalition of the besieged. For long periods of European history, Islam and Christianity were quite literally at each other's throats. The first time I visited Vienna, my hosts thought it important to take me to the hill that was the nearest the Ottoman Turks had got to the city walls during the Great Siege of 1683 (itself a re-run of the Turks' previous effort in 1529). Like Blücher and the Prussians at Waterloo, King John Sobieski and his Polish legions turned up at the last moment to ensure the Sultan's defeat. In 1699, the Treaty of Carlowitz marked the beginning of the end for Turkey's attempt to conquer Europe for Islam. In the south, the Iberian Muslim empire got as far as Poitiers in 732 before being defeated and permanently sent back beyond the Pyrenees by Charles Martel. As for Judaism, the history of Christian anti-semitism (for until the rise of Zionism, it had hardly any institutional existence in non-Christian countries) is long and extremely murderous.

Yet we now see leading Christian, Islamic and Jewish clerics getting into the same bed to protest against the wicked arguments of unbelievers who reject the central, fundamental idea of a god, because that threatens all of them, however much they still believe that the other creeds are mistaken or dangerously heretical. Officially, Roman Catholicism believes that even the Archbishop of Canterbury and his fellow bishops and archbishops will not get to heaven or will, at most, only be admitted to seats with a restricted view, let alone the various Muftis, Imams and Ayatollahs; or the Chief Rabbi. Many Muslim scholars, citing the Koran, do not accept Christianity's most fundamental claims; that Jesus was the son of God, as opposed to his servant and messenger, and suffered and died on the cross for our sins.[247] In the House of Lords, the 26 bishops of the Church of England who still have guaranteed seats and votes in our second chamber, actively seek the support of Catholic, Jewish and Muslim peers to block legislation that they believe to be against the will of God. Genetic manipulation to prevent lethal inheritable mitochondrial diseases and allowing dying patients to choose the time and manner of their deaths are among recent proposals that they jointly opposed.

History provides many examples of (relatively) good people having to work with and support some very bad people in the interests of national or mutual survival. The principle that 'my enemy's enemy is my friend' is often justified in the short term, however ghastly the new friend, but it may end in tears. As is now quite widely known, thanks to a 2007 film, the release of some (though not all) of the relevant Soviet documents and the tragic crash of an airliner carrying several dozen prominent Poles to a commemoration of the event, the Katyn massacre almost caused a serious rift between the Western Allies and the Soviet Union when it was revealed in 1943. In that year, Nazi troops uncovered mass graves containing the bodies of thousands of Polish officers and other leading Polish citizens who had all been shot in the head. It was clear from evidence at the site that the men had been killed in 1940 and the site was in the area of Eastern Poland that the Soviets had annexed after the Nazi-Soviet pact of August 1939, well before the Nazis invaded Russia in mid-1941. Goebbels made the most of it. An international body of forensic experts, including several from neutral countries, backed up the Nazi claim.

Had the Polish bodies been discovered before Hitler invaded Russia and when the Soviet Union was still officially an ally of the Nazis, Churchill would presumably have denounced it as yet another example of Soviet barbarity, to go with the Show Trials and the Ukrainian famine of the 1930s. Few non-communists in the West believed the hurried and unconvincing Soviet denials but Russia was now our gallant and strategically vital ally, so we had to go along with the Soviet version, backed up with hastily forged evidence, that the killing had taken place *after* mid-1941. At the Nuremberg war-crime trials in 1946, the USSR even had the cheek to try to get the Katyn massacre included in the charges against the Nazis. Subsequent attempts to erect a memorial in London to the victims of Stalinism were strongly discouraged for many years by British governments anxious not to upset Moscow more than necessary. Only after the USSR imploded was the truth gradually admitted by the post-Soviet authorities, or unearthed by the new breed of Russian historians during the few years when they had some access to the KGB archives.

Ideology and the politics of survival combined to block attempts to get at the truth. Public disbelief had to be minimized because over 90% of all the German military dead in the last two years of the war were killed by Russians, not by the Western allies. Today, leading Christian, Islamic and Jewish clerics in Western countries do not often publicly criticise the fundamental tenets of each other's religions because in secular societies, two can play at that game. In much the same way, the equivalent factions in CAM are reluctant to criticise, expose or even mention what many of them feel are untruths because to do so would threaten the greater good of defending CAM against its critics. Their enemy's enemy is their friend and that may be more important than the facts; or their patients.

Not all members of particular religions or sects welcome this sort of ecumenical love-in, even when it is politically expedient. *Catholic Family News,* 'a monthly journal preserving our Catholic faith and heritage', deplored the 2014 visit of Pope Francis to the Blue Mosque in Istanbul, during which he appeared to be actually *praying.* "This action defies Catholic Tradition, spurns the perennial Papal doctrine against religious indifferentism, and mocks true Catholics such as St. Francis of Assisi who visited Muslims for one purpose alone, to convert them to Christ's one true Church." I had not realised that St Francis, after whom the last pope named himself, was so intolerant when it came to heresy but it seems he was only obeying orders. The story continues: "At the Council of Carthage held in the year 398, at which Saint Augustine was present, the Church declares: 'None must either pray or sing psalms with heretics; and whosoever shall communicate with those who are cut off from the Communion of the Church, whether clergyman or laic, let him be excommunicated'. (Coun. Carth. iv. 72 and 73)".[248]

Those attitudes are still quite common in many parts of the world. The more traditional state of affairs was nicely (if unintentionally) captured by veteran war correspondent, Christopher Hedges, when he found that during the Yugoslav conflicts of the 1990s, "The clerics, on all three sides [i.e. Serbian Orthodox, Catholic and Muslim] were a disgrace. U.N. mediators in Sarajevo wearily complained that it was easier to get [military] commanders to the table for talks than the opposing clerics".[249] Perhaps the same uncompromising stance is taken by some CAM practitioners. After all, if – like Samuel Hahnemann - you truly believe that "There could not possibly be any true, best way of curing ... diseases other than pure homoeopathy", I can imagine that you might not want to be seen rubbing shoulders with riff-raff like acupuncturists, chiropractors, crystal healers and aromatherapists.

Chapter 18
Psychoanalysis explains everything...
...and the missing word in Freud's index

During the mid-1960s, Barbara Wootton, one of the most influential British sociologists, predicted that a century or two hence, we would all be influenced more by Freud than by Jesus. Psychoanalysis was still a powerful force in British psychiatry at that time but nothing like as powerful as it was in the USA. In the leading US journals of the period, like the *American Journal of Psychiatry* and *Archives of General Psychiatry,* sometimes half the papers in an individual issue invoked concepts and theories of a broadly psychoanalytic nature. Within a decade, papers like that were either not being submitted to the leading psychiatric journals or were being rejected. There were certainly good reasons for rejection, given the increasing requirement for evidence to support therapeutic claims but ultimately, it was due to the personality and therapeutic arrogance of the founder of psychoanalysis. Like Samuel Hahnemann, Sigmund Freud was self-deluding, grandiose, dogmatic and utterly convinced of the brilliance and correctness of his ideas. In May 1913, he wrote: "We possess the truth; I am as sure of it as fifteen years ago",[250] a chronology that takes us back to 1898 when Freud had barely finished creating the basic concepts of psychoanalysis. My main focus here is on the similarities between psychoanalysis and religion as healing ideologies and rituals but some remarkable features of that creative process are also worth recounting. An additional reason for including psychoanalysis is to demonstrate its unsuitability for helping us to understand placebo effects. Freud never seems to have considered them but even if he had, psychoanalysis would not be a reliable guide to the psychological processes that mediate placebo effects, because it is not a reliable guide to any aspect of human psychology and behaviour. Very few psychiatrists and even fewer medical scientists now share Freud's certainty that 'we possess the truth'.

Freud's admirers, who are still numerous and influential though now mostly outside psychiatry, regularly claim that he was ahead of his time and that he was a scientist as well as a healer. Some of them may now be happy to see him as just another philosopher but when Freud was developing the ideas that eventually culminated in psychoanalysis, it is very clear that he saw it purely as a technique for treating and curing the patients he had begun to see in *fin-de-siècle* Vienna. If psychoanalysis had not been widely promoted from the outset as a highly effective treatment, it would surely never have achieved the prominence and influence that it did. That it was demanding in terms of time and money and could be emotionally painful made it seem a kind of pilgrimage, though nobody at the time – least of all Freud himself – considered the very large placebo and non-specific effects of involvement in purposeful, disciplined and demanding activity that are among the benefits of pilgrimages. Psychoanalysis did not literally involve sore feet and muscles or long and perilous journeys through brigand-infested mountains but those traumatic memories – real or, as several 'false memory' cases have shown, imagined or induced – had to be delivered in quasi-obstetric pain and messiness through a psychoanalytic birth-canal and without anaesthesia, let alone the psychotherapeutic equivalent of a Caesarean section for those too emotionally posh to push.

The therapeutic claims and theories of psychoanalysis are similar to those of religion but the schisms and ferocious arguments that have characterised the first century of the Freudian era are also reminiscent of the theological debates, anathematisations and mutual excommunications of early Christianity.[251] One of the most important recent historians of psychoanalysis is Jeffrey Moussaieff Masson, who trained as an analyst after a period of psychoanalytic treatment. (The tendency of patients of analysts to become therapists subsequently is similar to the way in which former residents in clinics based exclusively on the doctrines of Alcoholics Anonymous are encouraged to become therapists.) Whatever we think of psychoanalysis, few people will disagree with Massons's claim that "...more has been written about [Freud] than about any other thinker of our time, probably because he did so much to alter the contours of the emotional and intellectual age in which we all live."

Freud's closest friend and intellectual collaborator at the time when he was developing his basic ideas was another emancipated Jewish doctor of a similar age, Wilhelm Fliess. Unlike Freud, Fliess was not a psychiatrist or neurologist: he was primarily an Ear, Nose and Throat (ENT) surgeon. Between 1887 and 1904, Freud wrote many letters to Fliess and received many in return. He also quite often visited the German-born Fliess in Berlin, where he practised. Most of the letters written to Freud by Fliess have not survived but 284 letters to Fliess from Freud have been preserved. Freud learned of their existence a year or two before his death from mouth cancer was pre-empted by his medically-assisted suicide in 1939. (Sometimes, a cigar is only a cigar, as Freud famously quipped, but it can still be lethally carcinogenic.) He was not pleased about their discovery, even though the letters had been obtained with difficulty by Princess Marie Bonaparte, a former patient who later became an analyst and was one of his most prominent supporters. This feisty woman had made the mistake of temporarily depositing the letters in the Rothschild Bank in Vienna in 1937 shortly before the Nazis marched in but managed to get them out again under the gaze of the Gestapo, after the *Anschluss* in 1938. Marie Bonaparte also had some interesting ideas of her own about the importance, for orgasmic purposes, of the distance between the clitoris and the vaginal opening. Her own orgasms were unsatisfactory and as a 'téléclitoridienne', she therefore had her clitoris surgically moved closer to her vagina. When this didn't produce the desired effect, she had it moved closer still. An exhibit in the Vienna Freud museum illustrated her theory with anatomical drawings and measurements precise to the nearest millimetre. Another described her therapeutic style as "…unorthodox, taking place in the garden in fair weather, with Bonaparte crocheting while she listens. Her chauffeur collects the patients and drives them back".

How perceptive Fliess's widow was when she specified that as a condition of sale, the letters should never come into Freud's hands, for he would almost certainly have destroyed them, as he may have destroyed most of the letters he received from Fliess. Freud told Marie Bonaparte that he wanted the letters burned but Freud's typically ideological habit of cooking the history books had appeared much earlier. Adam Phillips, one of Freud's most prominent current British defenders, records without any hint of censure that the 35-year-old Freud not only destroyed all papers and letters relating to his professional development but also made it clear that "we have no desire to make it too easy for [biographers]". Phillips adds – again uncritically – that at 35, "Freud thinks of himself as a hero, a man who will be worthy not of one biography but of many".[252] Fortunately for historians, Marie Bonaparte refused to destroy them but when the letters were eventually published in the 1950s, only 168 of the 284 were included and from many of those, large sections were deleted, often without any indication that possibly important passages had been removed. After reading them and learning more about some of Fliess's own theories, one can see why the Freudian apostles might have used their blue pencils rather vigorously and history should thank Masson for restoring the missing letters and passages.

There are several reasons why Freud might have wanted to burn the Fliess letters, as he had burned his earlier documents. It would be nice to think they included a belated realisation that if they were published, they would show him to have been, at heart, foolish, credulous, vain and wrong. When Masson became, for a while, the director of the Freud Archives in New York, he found that some files were marked 'not to be opened for a hundred years'. He ignored this anti-scientific and anti-historiographical instruction because it seemed that "a great many of the documents were kept from public view if, in the eyes of [the former director] or the donor, they could prove potentially embarrassing to psychoanalysis".[253] And also because, in spite of Freud's psychoanalyst daughter Anna's direct plea not to publish certain previously-suppressed or newly-discovered passages, Masson "felt that these passages not only were of great historical importance but might well represent the truth. *Nobody, it seemed to me, had the right to decide for others, by altering the record, what was truth and what was error".* [my italics] These attempts by Anna Freud and others to distort and suppress the early history of psychoanalysis have parallels in the rewriting of early Christian documents by copyists, the selection of only some of the numerous 'testaments' for the final form of the New Testament and the exclusion of certain other 'testaments' that conflicted with the preferred narrative that has been handed down to us.[254, 255] Just as Bishop Athanasius, in 367, ordered that "all gospels not included in his canon ... should be rooted out and destroyed",[256] the Koran is traditionally said to have achieved its present form only after the caliph Uthman's imposition of one particular compilation of Mohammed's revelations and the burning of the numerous competing versions. Dispassionate academic examination of the origins of the Bible began early in the 19th century but "the Islamic world", as Tom Holland, a respected historian of the period, delicately explains "has not, it is fair to say, shown any great inclination to follow suit". In a footnote criticising the popular religious historian Karen Armstrong, Holland also notes: "Remarkably for a book [about Islam] written by someone who has written extensively about the grand tradition of biblical scholarship, it does not so much as mention the problematic nature of the sources for the life of Muhammad". He also mentions the expulsion from Cairo University in the 1990s of Dr. Nasr Abu Zayd, a Koranic scholar, for mildly querying received opinion about the origins of the Koran. He was forced to divorce his wife and had to leave the country of his birth. [257]

Masson found a letter from the prominent psychoanalyst Otto Fenichel, which instructed that when an analytic institute "investigated a senior analyst for any infraction of medical conduct, this information should not be made public, lest it damage the credibility of psychoanalysis".[258] That is identical to the efforts of some religious institutions and senior clerics, notably in the Roman Catholic church and reaching as high as former popes, to conceal evidence of sexual wrongdoing by priests, a deception whose failure (and subsequent compensation cases) has bankrupted several Catholic dioceses around the globe. The religious overtones of psychoanalysis also emerge in another of Masson's discoveries. "It is not, in fact, uncommon for analysts to solicit, usually through roundabout methods, former patients for money to support analytic projects.'[259] Spontaneous donations from patients are one thing, though it can still be ethically questionable for psychiatrists in particular to accept them but to Masson (and to me) actively soliciting them is a very different thing and generally wrong. Yet although it is evidently common, Masson asks; 'Has any analyst of note ever objected to this publicly? I know of none". This is dangerously near to the sale of indulgences or the encouragement of rich parishioners to endow a chantry where masses might be said in perpetuity to ensure a place in heaven for their departed souls.

As the critic Frank Cioffi said about psychoanalysis following the collapse of yet another pillar of the Freudian temple: "In an ideal world, this would have knocked several more nails in Freud's coffin, but since it is so widely believed that he is not in it, having climbed out on the third day, it has had little discernible effect."[260] Masson concludes that "A psychoanalyst makes, ultimately, the same claims as a religious leader, and they are equally false. In my experience, psychoanalysis demands loyalty that could not be questioned, the blind acceptance of unexamined 'wisdom'. It is characteristic of religious orders to seek obedience without scepticism, but it spells the death of intellectual enquiry. All variants of 'because I say so' or because the Koran says so, or the Bible says so, or the Upanishads say so, or Freud says so, or Marx says so, are simply different means of stifling intellectual dissent."[261]

Therapeutic 'Grand Theories' may be particularly attractive to the sort of people who find grand religious or political theories persuasive and comforting; or who have apostasised from them and need an alternative. That might help to explain the curious co-existence of Marxist and Freudian ideologies in the same people, as with the philosopher Louis Althusser. Despite their incompatibilities, both ideologies dangled before their adherents the enticing possibility of a world in which major political, class or economic conflicts were reduced or abolished and a parallel therapeutic world in which unhappiness, overt insanity and disabling internal conflicts might also be, if not abolished, at least minimised.

Ironically, Freud recognised and criticised the similarities between Marxism and god-religions but failed to recognise that very similar criticisms could be made of psychoanalysis. "Any critical examination of Marxist theory", Freud wrote disapprovingly "is forbidden, doubts of its correctness are punished in the same way as heresy was once punished by the Catholic Church. The writings of Marx have taken the place of the Bible and the Koran as a source of revelation, though they would seem to be no more free from contradictions and obscurities than those older sacred books".[262] As the psychotherapist Anthony Storr comments, "If we substitute the word 'psychoanalysis' for 'Marxist theory' in the first sentence ... and the name 'Freud' for that of 'Marx' in the second sentence, we have an exact description of what happened to psychoanalysis ... *but Freud was unable to see this*". (my emphasis) For a man whose life's work was aimed at helping patients to become aware of repressed conflicts and events that supposedly impaired their ability to deal with reality, that is a very damning criticism. Storr regards Freud as a good example of a guru or cult-leader, along with people like Carl Jung and Rudolf Steiner. Typically, gurus are charismatic people; good writers and public speakers convinced that they have discovered truths denied to more ordinary mortals and that these truths are beyond question.

Freud was certainly a good writer and speaker and was unsuccessfully nominated for Nobel prizes in literature as well as medicine. Is it possible that some of the attraction that many people feel towards religion, homoeopathy, herbalism or psychoanalysis derives from the colourful and emotive language that suffuses their Sacred Texts? No good scientific paper describing the patients most likely to respond to, say, a drug for asthma would ever include such rhapsodic homoeopathic effusions as: "They are thirstless children who hate fat and like sweet things...and at night will sleep with their arms above their heads" without providing evidence for the claim. Cognitive behavioural therapy generally competes successfully with psychoanalysis when it comes to therapeutic effectiveness but its dry and meticulous chroniclers cannot hope to compete for literary style with a canon that includes phrases such as the *vagina dentata,* penis envy, the Oedipus complex, the collective unconscious, the madonna-prostitute split, castration anxiety and the good breast, that have some of the resonance (and helpful imprecision) of transubstantiation, the Holy Ghost, purgatory and predestination. Truly, the Devil has all the best tunes.

There is another and rarely-discussed similarity between organised Freudianity and organised Christianity and that is in the attitudes to homosexuality in their respective priesthoods, among both of which groups it is probably over-represented compared with the general public. For the last half-century, the Church of England especially has been publicly torturing itself by trying and failing to reconcile the circle of diversity and tolerance with the uncompromising square of sexual orthodoxy in the Old and New Testaments. In both institutions, this leads to a fascinating gamut of compromises, deceptions, self-deceptions and hypocrisies, ranging from marriages of convenience to a gay Pope (Julius III) who made his rent-boy a cardinal. Until barely a generation ago, it was uncommon for an openly gay clergyman or clergywoman to run a parish and it is still the official position of both Rome and Canterbury that priests who allow their yearnings (which are reluctantly permitted) to become genital acts (which are not) should expect little promotion, if indeed they get as far as ordination. Like the Church of England, the Church of Psychoanalysis did not officially admit gay trainees to the various seminaries that formed a kind of cathedral precinct around the Institute of Psychoanalysis and the Tavistock Clinic at the foot of Fitzjohn's Avenue, an easy downhill walk from Freud's last residence in Hampstead. (A residence, incidentally, that his psychoanalyst daughter, Anna, shared until her death with fellow-psychoanalyst Dorothy Burlingham in what was very obviously a lesbian relationship.) Freudianity may have changed the rules by now. A related similarity is that just as the shortage of British-born ordinands has led to the presence of many Anglicans and Catholics from other countries and continents in British training colleges for the clergy, so have the Freudians had to admit many more trainee analysts from overseas because of a shortage of indigenous acolytes. The would-be priests come mainly from Africa. Many would-be psychoanalysts come from Eastern Europe, where they may have ditched Communism but not, alas, –isms in general, a point recently confirmed by two sceptical Polish psychologists.[263] There is also a sizeable contingent from South America, where Freudo-Marxism flourishes.

Masson's personal history is typical of a certain kind of person who ends up 'in therapy'. His parents, though kind, loving and not at all abusive in any of the usual senses of the word, graduated *summa cum laude* from the Philip Larkin school of child-rearing.[264] He was born in

Chicago in 1941 into an intense, cosmopolitan and vegetarian Jewish family who were close to, and heavily influenced by, Paul Brunton (1898-1981) a charismatic British mystic and – as it turned out – a total fraud. He claimed to have been a Tibetan and to have lived on Venus in previous incarnations and, says Masson, 'At twelve, it never occurred to me to be sceptical'.[265] During a family outing on a Hawaiian beach, this pubescent credulity and arrogance led him to dismiss a mundane question from his younger sister thus: 'Woman, I have just been reading *The Mysterious Kundalini* and cannot be disturbed in my contemplations'. (To which she sensibly if precociously replied 'What bullshit!'.)[266] When Masson asked Brunton why he didn't have a driving licence, he explained that on Venus, there were no cars. Later, when Masson studied Sanskrit, he discovered that Brunton had completely misinterpreted some important ancient Hindu texts; and that Brunton's claim to be fluent in Sanskrit was as false as his claim to have a PhD from a reputable US university. This experience turned out to be useful and very relevant when he came to study the guru's psychoanalytic equivalents. However, it has to be admitted that in both cases, the scales took a long time to fall from Masson's eyes.

Before they did so, Masson had an encounter with a visiting Indian philosophy professor and guru in her forties who had invited a few followers to her apartment. During the discussion, she claimed that her mind was entirely filled with spiritual thoughts to the exclusion of fleshly ones. As the guests were leaving, she asked young Masson – still attractive in his 70s when I interviewed him - to stay behind "as there was something she wanted to tell me". Here is Masson's description of the events that followed.

> Lady Guru: 'You don't believe I am free of sexual desire?'
> Young Masson: 'No'.
> LG: 'I will prove it to you. Touch my breasts'.
> Masson did as he was told.
> 'See, I feel nothing. Now touch my thighs'.
> Masson obliged.
> LG. 'Again, nothing. Even if you enter me with your penis, I will feel nothing. Do you believe me?'
> YM: 'No'.
> LG: 'Try'.
> He did.
> LG: 'See, I feel nothing sexual. The whole time this is going on I am thinking only about the higher self, the *atman*'.[267]

This is an unusually credible and well-documented example of how clerics and gurus use their spiritual authority to take sexual advantage of their credulous and – in Masson's case – sexually and socially inexperienced followers, but it's evidently an old trick. In *Risorgimento* Italy, there were many sweaty couplings among the nuns of Sant 'Ambrogio in Rome and between the nuns and their male clerical visitors and confessors. One of these, the theologian, philosopher and Jesuit Joseph Kleutgen, later assured an investigating judge that when he was French kissing a young, beautiful and aristocratic novice – an activity that the Vatican then prohibited as "sinfully lustful" even among married couples – "his thoughts flowed upwards to God".[268]

A Harvard student and extremely bright, young Masson quickly became professor of Sanskrit at Toronto University. This is not an obvious route of entry into psychoanalysis but Masson explains and he is much more forthcoming about his own early life than Freud was about his. Unsurprisingly, young Jeffrey was not a happy man.[269] One misty autumn evening in Harvard, he got lost and knocked on the door of a brightly-lit house, which happened to belong to a husband-and-wife pair of psychoanalysts, the first of that genus that Masson had ever met. They were friendly and open, as academics and professionals in university towns usually are towards students. He had been 'lonely at Harvard' and 'unable to fall in love'. Masson warmed to their 'kindly intimacy' and wanted more of it; he yearned for 'the connection with another human soul'.[270] They suggested that he 'might be interested in therapy'. Well, I suppose they would say that.

After an unhelpful encounter with conventional psychiatry, he married a survivor of the Warsaw ghetto who was having psychoanalysis. Despite the marriage, he still felt afflicted with "an almost congenital sadness. I was convinced that psychoanalysis would have the answers to my personal unhappiness". He completed a training analysis (a damaging and depressing experience, as he describes it) and subsequently became accredited as a practising psychoanalyst. Later, he was fiercely critical of 'this "men's club" with its initiation rites; expectations of membership loyalty over truth; pressures to accept concepts handed down by the leader, no matter how irrational; xenophobic banding together against outsiders; and the punishment of anyone who poses questions or finally wants out.' However, at that stage, he was as enthusiastic about Freud and psychoanalysis as he had once been about Brunton and Indian mythology and he soon turned on it the full and formidable force of his academic talents. His youthful energy and charm impressed an old Middle European refugee psychoanalyst called Kurt Eissler, who had found sanctuary from the Nazis in New York. Eissler had also become the guardian of the extensive Freud archives where mainly documentary relics and memorabilia of Freud were stored. To this treasure-chamber, Masson was literally given the keys. Since Masson was not only young, bright and energetic but also a fellow-admirer of The Master, Eissler thought that he was a safe pair of hands even for documents that might be rather compromising. Like the Fliess correspondence. For a while, Masson even succeeded him as Director of the Archives.

Partly in order to read these venerable (and venerated) documents in the original, Masson added fluent German to his already impressive linguistic repertoire, spending some time in Munich in the process. After initially welcoming him, the psychoanalysts of that city later excommunicated him in a manner very reminiscent of the ways in which the Spanish Inquisition and Soviet psychiatry suppressed dissidents. Always the eager and dedicated academic, Masson presented a paper to a meeting of his fellow-analysts about Sandor Ferenczi, one of Freud's original circle who, in the last year or two of his life, fell out with him on an important clinical and theoretical point. Their disagreement concerned the truth or otherwise of claims by patients that they had been sexually abused in childhood, an issue that is still very much with us and one that can obviously be difficult to verify in an individual case. Ferenczi had disagreed with Freud on this point. Masson's paper supported Ferenczi. After he had finished, one of his new Munich friends, who supported the orthodox Freudian position, stood up: "I don't know how to say this but I feel forced to say that you are dangerously mentally ill. In fact, Jeff, I believe you should spend some time in a psychiatric hospital [and] I am prepared to commit you tonight if one of the gentlemen in the room will second my opinion".[271] Masson thought he was joking. He wasn't. Most of the others were also deeply offended by Masson's heresy, though fortunately not to the point of dragging poor Jeff off to the local mad-house. The subsequent ferocious debate that followed the publication of Masson's *The Assault on Truth* is not relevant to this chapter. In that book, he argued, like Ferenczi, that many 'neurotic' patients had experienced real sexual abuse, as Freud originally claimed, and were not simply fantasizing about sexual encounters and desires, as posited by Freud and psychoanalysis in its developed form. Masson also argued that Freud's change of mind was strongly influenced by the disapproval of colleagues and the catastrophic results, described shortly, of letting Fliess operate on one of Freud's patients.

Masson wasn't content with simply publishing the missing letters and the suppressed paragraphs that he found in his new realm. He befriended Freud's ageing daughter Anna and she eventually gave him the run of the house in Maresfield Gardens, Hampstead – now the Freud Museum - where Freud had lived after his exile from Vienna and where she remained after Freud died until her own death in 1982. He gives us this revealing vignette. 'There was a purity of purpose, a holiness to her devotion [to psychoanalysis] that gave off a whiff of religious piety...I am sure she got [this trait] from her father, who of course was entirely consumed with holy zeal for the cause'.[272] The house contained not only Freud's extensive and eclectic library, with his many pencilled marginal comments, but also several additional letters from Fliess and unpublished correspondence with other leading figures in the development of psychoanalysis. Masson put all this detective work to good use in *The Assault on Truth* but at that time, he was still convinced of the basic validity and therapeutic effectiveness of psychoanalysis. Disenchantment came several years later. Meanwhile, he published the first complete and unexpurgated version of the letters.[273]

They show that as well as discussing his theories with Fliess, Freud also felt extremely close to him personally and emotionally. Often, the salutation of early letters is 'Dearest Friend' or just 'Dearest'. One letter that would turn out to be particularly important in the history of psychoanalysis continues: "Why don't you write? How are you? Don't you care any more about what I am doing?" but then continues: "What is happening to the nose, menstruation, labour pains, neuroses, your dear wife and the budding little ones?".

"The nose, menstruation, labour pains, neuroses" just about sums up their areas of common medical concern at that time. For an ENT surgeon to be interested in noses is, of course, unremarkable but 'menstruation, labour pains, neuroses' as well? Fliess, it seems, was no ordinary ENT surgeon. Who egged on whom is not entirely clear, though it is likely that Fliess was the dominant partner. What is clear is that both of them were obsessed with the idea of sex as the motor that drives not just some but all human thought and activity, including "the neuroses". It certainly became a fundamental tenet of psychoanalytic theory, as a future US authority on addiction recalled being told in the mid-20th century during one of his undergraduate lectures.

"Chentlemen, zere is nussing to life but sex und aggression, und ze sooner you recognize zat, ze better".[274]

These notions incorporated common Victorian beliefs about the harmful effects of masturbation but Fliess had some theories of his own, chief among which was the 'nasal reflex neurosis'. According to Fliess, the nose contained important nerve connections to the rest of the body and in particular, to the genitalia. This led him to the *therapeutic* idea that by using the newly-discovered cocaine to anaesthetise these nasal 'G-spots' – to use a later but unscientific term - several disorders and discomforts could be relieved or cured. Following the old and noble but not always commendable medical tradition of doctors testing out their theories on themselves, as Hahnemann had done, Fliess spent quite a bit of time shoving cocaine-soaked swabs up his nose. He may not have known it but cocaine is rapidly absorbed from the nasal mucous membranes. Not surprisingly, Fliess felt better after these applications. Not surprisingly – since cocaine typically produces a sense of well-being and confidence – he interpreted this relief as further proof of the correctness of his theory. And not surprisingly, his dearest friend Sigmund joined him in these experiments, for Freud was a bit of a hypochondriac – a tendency not helped by his addiction to cigars, which may have caused heart problems before it probably caused his mouth cancer.

Most people who ever use cocaine do not subsequently have serious problems with it. That's true of almost the entire population of the Andean *altiplano* who have used it for several thousand years as a stimulant, albeit in less concentrated forms. However, it is significant that a disproportionate number of the victims of the first cocaine epidemic in the two or three decades around the end of the 19th century were physicians, including one of the greatest names in American surgery: William Halstead. Freud soon became rather fond of the stuff but unlike Halstead, he never had to be taken away by the men in white coats and incarcerated for three weeks in a yacht belonging to one of his colleagues to force him to break the habit: and neither did Freud abandon cocaine only to become, like Halstead, a well-functioning morphine addict instead. However, just as one of the symptoms of Halstead's problem was that he wrote page after page of high-flown nonsense, so the suspicion remains that at least some of Freud's writings during his crucial friendship with Fliess owed quite a lot to cocaine's energising and euphoriant effects. There is even a technical term to describe the literary consequences of cocaine use: *graphomania.*

Fliess's belief (and Freud's) in the nasal reflex neurosis meant that he was frequently doing things to Freud's nose, for Fliess believed that if applying cocaine to the 'G spots' didn't relieve symptoms, the next step was to cauterise (i.e. chemically burn) the spot or even to excise it, together with the delicate underlying turbinate bone if necessary. It is likely that the repeated cocainisations and cauterisations of Freud's nose led to a state of chronic inflammation and infection, which duly became the justification for further cocaine applications but it is clear that Freud also used cocaine deliberately for its mood-altering effects as well as its nose-altering ones. Here he is in May 1893:

"…a short time ago, I interrupted (for one hour) a severe migraine of my own with cocaine: the effect set in only after I had cocainised the opposite side as well; but then it did so promptly".

In April 1895:

"Today I can write because I have more hope; I pulled myself out of a miserable attack with a cocaine application. I cannot guarantee that I shall not come for a day or two for a cauterisation…"

In June, he writes:

"I am feeling I to IIa. [i.e. on some notional scale of happiness or health: I = low] I need a lot of cocaine."

Freud was sufficiently convinced by Fliess's view that 'G spots' should, if necessary, be excised that he let Fliess operate on one of his 'neurotic' patients, Emma Eckstein, who by that time had become a psychoanalyst herself. The results were disastrous and nearly fatal, and she spent much of the next ten years as an invalid until her death aged 59. Fliess somehow left a length of gauze packing inside the nasal cavity. Whether or not this was the cause, Emma bled profusely and repeatedly and for more than a week, Freud feared she would bleed to death. It was nearly three months before the bleeding and infection finally settled and her pain was severe enough to require frequent doses of morphine despite Freud's concern that she might become dependent on it. However, he then had the nerve to claim that "…her episodes of bleeding were hysterical…and probably occurred at the sexually relevant times…". (26th April 1896) He also persuaded himself that the surgery on her nose had not affected her appearance although her niece Ada Elias, a paediatrician, later wrote that "As a result, her face was disfigured—the bone was chiselled away, and on one side caved in."[275]

An explanation is needed for that otherwise puzzling phrase *"…probably occurred at the sexually relevant times"*. Fliess's other preoccupations included a belief that all human activity was controlled by

28-day or 23-day cycles. Freud at one stage tried to incorporate this idea into his own theories. 'I then note that I can account for all psychic periods as multiples of 23-day periods (π) if I *include in the calculation the period of gestation* (276 days = $12\,\pi$)' (6 December 1896, italics in original.) But as Masson notes: "The truth is that the source of her bleeding was to be found not in a series of 23-day and 28-day cycles nor in hysterical longing, but in an unnecessary operation which was performed because of a *folie à deux* on the part of two misguided doctors".[276]

Both of Fliess's cherished theories seem to be groundless and worthless so what are we to make of Freud's obvious enthusiasm for them? A *Times Literary Supplement* review of Masson's compilation cited on the book's cover refers to "the personal dynamics of one of the great acts of cultural creation in history as Freud produced what was to become a towering imaginative structure". Imagination has an important and honoured place in the production of scientific theory. (The centenary of Kekulé's famous dream about a circle of snakes each biting the tail of the snake in front, which led him to theorise how six carbon atoms could form a benzene ring, occasioned a commemorative British postage stamp.) Nevertheless, the acid test is whether the theory is eventually supported by the facts. There is no evidence that Freud seriously considered the possible placebo and non-specific effects of just talking and listening to patients, or of confession, and his claim that "Obsessional neurosis can be cured if we undo all the substitutions and affective transformations that have taken place..." (1st Jan 1896) is not observed in practice. Obsessive-Compulsive Disorder (OCD) is often rather resistant to treatment and if it responds to psychotherapy, the therapy most likely to be helpful is the cognitive-behavioural kind.

Freud's most famous OCD patient – the 'Wolf Man' – was a treatment failure, yet he has been written-up by Freudian disciples as a triumph.[277] By itself, a single case usually proves nothing – neither for nor against a particular treatment or theory – unless, like Freud, the promoters of the treatment in question are foolish enough to claim unfailing or even high effectiveness, but the Wolf Man story can tell us a lot about how Freud, in therapeutic rather than theoretical mode, viewed the effectiveness of the treatment that he was proud to have invented. In this case, unusually, we also know how the patient viewed it; and we know that both therapist and patient greatly overrated the success of the enterprise, though the patient eventually gained more insight into the failure than Freud or any of his subsequent therapists ever did.

To read Freud's own account of The Wolf Man is to enter a world in which unvalidated theory is treated as fact, possibilities are transmuted into probabilities or near-certainties and breath-taking assumptions about people he had never met are repeatedly made. This was a bad habit of Freud's. For example, although Freud never met the poet Ezra Pound, one of Pound's friends discussed his 'case' with Freud during her own psychoanalysis in 1933. Freud said that Pound had "very difficult Oedipal problems". That was arguably silly and arrogant enough but Freud then added that if he had known Pound, "I would have made him all right".[278] Since Pound was notoriously and publicly anti-Semitic for most of his life, that prediction is doubly questionable. Pound's equally notorious arrogance might also have made him reluctant to take advice from Freud, though shortly before he died, he had enough self-awareness to tell his fellow-poet Allen Ginsberg: "I started life with a swollen head. I'm ending it with swollen feet".

Wolf Man is important partly because the case gets its name from Freud's allegedly crucial interpretation of one of the patient's dreams and partly because it is one of the few analyses that Freud himself performed without soon handing over the case to one of his colleagues or students, though he did so later. However, it is also one of the very few analyses – perhaps the only one – in which really long-term and independent follow-up has been possible. Karin Obholzer, a young Viennese journalist, tracked the patient down sixty years after he was supposed to have been cured. She got to know him well, partly because despite four years of psychoanalysis from The Master, six days a week, and a further few months of treatment for some new manifestations of his basic obsessive-compulsive disorder, he still had serious difficulties in his relationships with women, which was one of the main problems that led him to consult Freud in the first place. With Obholzer, it seems that he could relax and talk in a way that he found impossible with most women and he evidently valued and enjoyed their meetings. For her part, Obholzer was sufficiently concerned for his welfare to keep visiting him even when he was admitted to a psychiatric hospital, where he became gradually demented and died aged 93.[279]

The Wolf Man - Sergei Konstantinovitch Pankeyev - was a rich young Russian from a family of minor aristocrats with a strong history of mental disturbance. Travelling around Europe just before the First World War, he became a sort of psychiatric tourist, starting in St Petersburg with the famous neuropsychiatrist Vladimir Bechterev, whose name is still attached to a leading research institute in that city. On some of his travels, he was accompanied by a medical student and by Dr. Leonid Drosnes, a physician who had treated him in Odessa and who first suggested that he consult Freud. The task of the medical student was to be an extra pair of hands for their card games and to administer the enemas that young Sergei's obsession with his bowels (among other obsessive-compulsive concerns) made a regular requirement. His mother was a hypochondriac. His father had episodes of depression and had consulted psychiatrists himself, in an age when psychiatric consultations were very much less common – and much more stigmatised – than they are today. One of his uncles – "an extreme case of misanthropy" – died in total and paranoid isolation on his remote estate. A paranoid maternal cousin "ended up in an insane asylum in Prague". A grandmother probably killed herself. His older sister Anna certainly did so (rather stylishly, while visiting the site of the poet Lermontov's fatal duel) thus precipitating Sergei's second breakdown. The first had occurred a year earlier, at eighteen, after he caught gonorrhoea. When he was 21, his father also killed himself. In Obholzer's understated words, "It cannot be surprising that with such a family background, a person should make a career of being a patient". Perhaps the real surprise is that he seems not to have seen a psychiatrist until he was eighteen.

In one of the private sanatoria where he was treated before seeing Freud, he fell in love with one of his nurses and eventually married her, though not until Freud – after four years of psychoanalysis – allowed him to do so. As one might guess, this union did not end happily. During the analysis, Sergei recounted the famous childhood dream that gave rise to his fame as The Wolf Man, in which he describes seeing six white wolves in the branches of a tree outside his bedroom window. For a Russian child of the late 19th century to dream of wolves is perhaps not very remarkable, frightening though it evidently was at the time, but in Freud's hands, the wolves become clear evidence of Oedipal and castration anxieties. Anxieties, furthermore, that arose not only from allegedly seeing, at the age of one and a half, his parents having sex in a classic 'primal scene' but having it, quite specifically, doggy-style ('*a tergo*' in Freud's coy Latin) and no less than three times during the same afternoon. The white wolves, according to Freud, represented the parents' white underwear.

After four years of psychoanalysis, Sergei was regarded by Freud as cured and returned to Russia shortly before WW1 started. In 1918, while in Bucharest, he learned that the Red Army had occupied Odessa and returned to Vienna where he soon visited Freud again. Freud recommended re-analysis because of a small "unanalysed residue". This lasted for about a year. Unable to return to Russia and now progressively deprived of his family's former riches, Sergei found work with a Viennese insurance company and stayed with them until he retired at 65. Soon after their marriage, his wife's daughter by her previous husband died. She and Sergei had no children but went for regular country walks at weekends while Sergei did a little landscape-painting. Having married a rich aristocrat, his wife did not adapt well to mere gentility and a few days after the 1938 *anschluss,* she joined the impressive list of suicides that had impinged on Sergei's life.

It would not be surprising if this blow made Sergei turn once again to psychoanalysis for help but he had already done so in 1926, when Freud referred him to one of his pupils, the American psychiatrist Ruth Mack Brunswick. She believed that during Freud's treatment, the 'transference' – simply put, the way the patient's childhood relationships influence the patient-therapist relationship – had not been sufficiently "lived through". Sergei, in fact, had moved on from an obsession with his bowels to a concern with his nose and his general appearance that at times bordered on the delusional. Brunswick regarded it as another manifestation of 'castration anxiety'. (Acupuncturists believe that needles cure diseases; psychoanalysts believe that interpretations do so.) Incidentally, although – as with Halstead and his cocaine problem – it does not necessarily reflect on her competence, the twice-divorced Brunswick became addicted to opiates and died aged only 48 after falling in her bathroom while intoxicated. The *American Journal of Psychoanalysis* – the house-journal of a profession that encouraged patients to be ruthlessly honest about even small details of their lives – wrote only that "She had a sudden tragic death".[280]

After WW2, another American psychoanalyst, Muriel Gardiner, met this famous patient, by then aged about seventy, thus beginning a final round of psychoanalysis that continued intermittently for the next decade or so. She reported: "The chief feature [of Sergei] is the prominence of his obsessional doubting, brooding ... completely engrossed in his own problems and unable to relate to others", yet she managed to persuade herself that "the positive results of the Wolf M-man's analysis are impressive indeed". Just how impressive they were, as Obholzer commented, "the reader will be able to judge for himself, once he has read the conversations that follow".

The God Effect

Among the many sad stories that old Sergei told young Karin, there are some very strange ones concerning his continuing contact with the world of psychoanalysis. An analyst in New York, identified only as 'E' (I think it very likely that he was Kurt Eissler, Masson's predecessor as Keeper of the Freud Archives) regularly sent Sergei money. What might seem like kindness to an old man – who occasionally sent 'E' one of his landscapes – was actually money that poor old Sergei needed not for himself but to fend off the demands of a younger Viennese woman who had become his unwelcome and unwanted companion. She demanded money for clothes and Sergei, who had always had difficulties in his relationships with women and was plagued by classic obsessional indecision, was unable to shake her off. This passage in Obholzers's book says it all:

> Obholzer. "So you actually get a kind of pension from the Freud archive?"
> Sergei. "...which does me no good, it's for the woman. If they sent it to me, and I kept it, I could live quite well".

Freud told young Sergei that if he had not become a psychoanalyst, he would have become an economist. That might be a troubling thought if there were not as many put-downs about economists as there are about psychoanalysts (such as JK Galbraith's quip that 'economic forecasting was invented to make astrology look good'). As to Freud's personal economic programme, his hourly rate was 40 Austro-Hungarian crowns. Comparisons of ancient and modern prices are not a simple matter and can be contradictory. For example, a US dollar was worth about five crowns in 1910 and a British pound would buy you about five dollars. £1.75 doesn't sound a lot for a consultation but a correspondent to the BMJ that year[281] complained that an insurance company expected him to do a home visit to a patient living three miles away and write a report for only half a (British) crown – about 12 pence (15 US or Euro-cents) in today's money. A better comparison, made by old Sergei himself, was that a day's in-patient care at 'a first-rate sanatorium' cost about 12 crowns. That was less than a third of what young Sergei paid for an hour of Freud's steamy imaginings at 9 Berggasse. In 2025, a day in a 'superior' room at a first-rate private psychiatric hospital in Britain would cost *more*, not less, than most private psychiatrists would charge for at least an hour's initial consultation and a detailed report to the referring GP.

Although it had a much happier long-term outcome, the case-history of another of Freud's famous patients has much in common with the story of the Wolf Man. Indeed, the patient might reasonably have been remembered as 'the Horse-Boy' but he has come down to us instead as 'Little Hans', the subject of Freud's 'Analysis of a phobia in a five-year-old boy'. Freud never actually 'analysed' Hans and the analysis was conducted at second-hand by Hans's father, a distinguished music critic and an enthusiastic convert to the Freudian faith. The four-year-old Hans was frightened when a horse drawing a heavily-laden cart collapsed very near him and he became a bit phobic about walking in streets in case the same thing happened again. Like most four-year-olds who develop phobias, Hans soon grew out of it and eventually followed his father into a successful career as a critic and opera producer. Naturally, for Freud and for Hans's father, Max, nothing could be that simple. (Psychoanalysts have their own version of Pope John-Paul II's claim that "in the designs of Providence, there are no mere coincidences".) The uninitiated and unconverted might think that Hans's short-lived fear of horses was basically just that – the understandable reaction of a child exploring the strange, exciting but sometimes frightening new world outside his familiar, domestic comfort-zone – but both Sigmund and Max saw in it the programmed and doctrinally pre-destined stirrings of infantile sexuality, though they differed as to which particular stirrings were involved. Max thought that his son's symptoms constituted displacement anxiety after being sexually excited by maternal caresses and the sight of the horse's penis. Freud thought that the recent addition to the family of a sister and the consequent sibling rivalry and Oedipal conflicts were crucial factors. He advised Max to explain the business of sex to little Hans and when Hans got better, he concluded – elephant-joke style – that this proved the correctness and usefulness of his advice. Not all the children of psychoanalysts and their fellow-travellers escape as lightly as Little Hans did. Nobody has done a systematic head-count and follow up but if someone ever did, I very strongly suspect that they would encounter much more than the expected number of unhappy and dysfunctional sons and daughters. Self-defined experts on child development are not necessarily successful parents.

Finally, that missing word in the Freudian index between 'penis' and 'pleasure' is, of course, 'placebo'.[282] Yet what Freud ignored was recognised in 1604 by King James I/VI in his famous *Counterblaste to tobacco*, when the newly-imported North American leaf was being touted as a cure-all, rather like psychoanalysis:

> "For is it not a very great mistaking, to take *non causam pro causa*, [i.e. wrongly attributing a cause] as they say in the Logicks? Because peradventure

when a sicke man hath had his disease at the height, hee hath at that instant taken Tobacco, and afterward his disease taking the naturall course of declining, and consequently the patient of recovering his health, O then the Tobacco forsooth, was the worker of that miracle. Beside that, it is a thing well knoweil to all Phisicians, that *the apprehension and conceit of the patient hath by wakening and uniting the vitall spirits, and so strengthening nature, a great power and vertue, to cure divers diseases. ...* and so if a man chance to recover one of any disease, after he hath taken Tobacco, that must have the thankes of all."[283] (my italics).

Chapter 19
But what do they know about placebos?
A friendly critique of Richard Dawkins, Daniel Dennett and Sam Harris

Like detailed research into the meaning and experience of placebo effects for individual patients, examining the similarities between religion and placebos is a very recent activity. I'm not the first person to note the similarity, and in his very readable *How God Works*[284], Prof David DeSteno has a few pages on it, but he confirmed that this book is its first discussion in depth and detail. In *The God Delusion*, Richard Dawkins mentioned the idea briefly[285] but he didn't develop it and neither, as far as I can see, did any of the other recent god-critics. It doesn't appear in the index of the popular religious critiques by Daniel Dennett, Sam Harris or Christopher Hitchens, excellent though they are in other respects. For Sam Harris not to mention the placebo effect is rather surprising, since he is a neuroscientist, though perhaps he has never worked much with clinicians or patients. It's not discussed by any of the 47 prominent sceptics from Lucretius and Spinoza to Philip Larkin in Hitchens's *A Portable Atheist*[286] subtitled 'Essential readings for the nonbeliever'. It's true that most of them died long before placebos were studied but King James and Thomas Sydenham can't have been the only sceptical early moderns.[287] The handful of bloggers who have mentioned the idea don't explore the wider implications and apart from DeSteno, neither does the only other academic discussion I can find.[288] Only the born-again American Christian and religious affairs journalist mentioned earlier, who described how "the placebo of faith ... had stopped working", seemed to be speaking from experience.[289]

That inevitable lack of clinical insight might explain why Dawkins underestimates the power of both positive and negative placebo and non-specific effects.[290] He does concede that "faith-healing might turn out to work in a few cases" and notes, correctly, that "it in no way boost[s] the truth value of religious claims" but placebo effects help very much more than "a few" patients. Dawkins also admits that he himself has often "been instantly 'cured' of some minor ailment by a reassuring voice from an intelligent face surmounting a stethoscope" but seems not to realise that even in serious illness, placebo effects can be extremely powerful, both subjectively and objectively, especially when psychological factors are an important part of the overall picture. Finally, Dawkins may not realise that placebo effects are not only real but also both measurable and measured.

For Dawkins, "the placebo theory [is] unworthy of the massively pervasive worldwide phenomenon of religion. I don't think the reason we have religion is that it reduced the stress levels of our ancestors. That's not a big enough theory for the job, although it may have played a subsidiary role". My view is that it played a lot more than that and the great 18th century philosopher (and probable atheist) David Hume agrees. He thought that "the first ideas of religion arose not from a contemplation of the works of nature, but from a concern with regard to the events of life, and from the incessant hopes and fears, which actuate the human mind". These fears included "the dread of future misery", presumably including misery caused by diseases, and "the terror of death".[291] Dawkins quotes Steven Pinker as saying 'pointedly' that "A freezing person finds no comfort in believing he is warm" but a person having his appendix removed under hypnosis clearly finds an enormous amount of comfort in being helped to believe that he is not feeling any pain and so - *pace* Pinker - does a hypnotized person immersed in ice-water. Part of my argument is that the powerful effects of hypnosis have some very important similarities to placebo effects in both medicine and religion.

Daniel Dennett was prepared to give some credit to the placebo effect's more dramatic manifestations as a factor in the evolution of shamanism but restricts the comparison mainly to obvious healing rituals, rather than to the many other ways in which religions, regardless of their doctrines and the truth or otherwise of their claims, can bring a variety of comforts to the afflicted. In citing a researcher who "hypothesize[s] that shamanic rituals constitute hypnotic inductions ... [and] that client responses are equivalent to responses produced by hypnosis",[292] Dennett supports my comparisons with hypnosis but largely ignores the much less dramatic everyday experiences of suggestion, hope, belief, faith and expectation that underlie the placebo effect. The ordinary suggestibility that is a built-in characteristic of humans and of several other animals does not need to match the extraordinary suggestibility of a hypnotic state to do its work. Finally, while many shamanic rituals were public, many of today's medical treatments, just like confession and several other religious activities, involve only the patient or parishioner and a single healer or priest. Indeed, neither the patient benefiting from the placebo effects of taking medication that contains no pharmacologically active ingredients, nor the parishioner praying quietly at home to a deity who doesn't exist or doesn't care, needs the real presence of another human to feel better. As always, 'the consolation of imaginary things is not imaginary consolation' and as mentioned previously, an advantage of religious placebos over the medical kind is that helpful habits of ritual and belief are usually instilled and normalised at an early age.

I am certainly not arguing that placebo and non-specific effects account *by themselves* for the phenomena of religious belief and behaviour. Like all the writers mentioned above, I regard religion – as we should surely regard all human activity – as multifactorial in its origins. However, I do argue that placebo effects are not only one of that multiplicity of factors but also an important and regularly under-estimated one. Those other factors include a variety of psychological and social processes that are not specifically linked to the placebo response and come under the general heading of 'psychology of religion'.[293] They also include neuropsychological and neurophysiological factors, both general and individual. All learning and all adaptation involves neuroanatomy – the various regions of the brain – and the chemical and physiological processes that enable those regions to perform their particular functions, to adapt to new experiences (neuroplasticity) and to communicate with other regions. The factors may also include evolutionary processes that made it easier for young mammals to find and interact with their mothers, thus improving their survivability and possibly explaining why many humans experience a 'sensed presence' that may be interpreted as contact with a god-figure.[294]

In *The Believing Brain* (subtitled; 'From spiritual faiths to political convictions: how we construct beliefs and reinforce them as truths') Michael Shermer reviews the main psychological mechanisms that mediate what he calls 'the cognitive biases of belief'. He discusses concepts like 'agenticity', 'patternicity' and 'confirmation bias' as well as specific dogmas such as belief in God, aliens, conspiracy theories and the afterlife that are often closely related to religious identification. These are valid and important points but Shermer also gives us a sentence from the novelist Upton Sinclair which, perhaps without his realizing it, summarises one of the important drivers of placebo effects – a concept that he does not mention. "It is difficult to get a man to understand something when his job depends on not understanding it". Placebo effects may have some of their origins in the difficulty of getting a man to understand that illness and dying are a normal part of life when, at some level, his peace of mind depends on preferring to think that they are not, or not in his case.

I noted earlier that religions are cultural, social, tribal, charitable and mutual support institutions, as well as purveyors of truth-claims about historical events, the purpose of existence, what the tribal deity wants from us during life and what happens to us after death, for example. These practical and social functions are extremely important and are another reason why churches can still flourish in countries like Denmark that have largely rejected the defining and often contradictory truth-claims. (As philosophers from antiquity onwards have pointed out, the contradictory claims of religions cannot all be true but they can certainly all be false.) I am mainly concerned here with one of those claims – the very important and frequently-invoked truth-claim that a named deity is able to prevent, relieve or cure illness and prevent or postpone a seemingly imminent death. As we have seen, it is an exaggeration to claim that 'there are no atheists in foxholes' but many people find themselves in the metaphorical foxhole of severe and life-threatening illness. They may be tempted to abandon or modify their religious doubts, and doubts about the quasi-religions of CAM.

Apart from their shared placebo and non-specific effects, there is one other point where medicine and religion combine in an intensely personal way that probably had little effect on the origins of religion *per se* but definitely had profound consequences for the history of particular religions and cults. The great psychologist William James called it 'religious fever', by which he meant the extremes of religious ecstasy, faith and feelings of personal connection with the relevant deity. These 'fevers' have been crucial for the origins of several sects. They may even have given rise to entire religions if the 'fever' and charisma of the founder happened to coincide with favourable events. As the writer and traveller Ryszard Kapuscinski noted:

> "The properties of a [social] structure are inertia, resilience and an amazing almost instinctive ability to survive. A structure is rather easy to create, and incomparably more difficult to destroy. *It can long outlast all the reasons that justified its establishment.*"[295] (my italics)

The economist Niall Ferguson was thinking of economic rather than religious evolution when he wrote:

> "Note that this may not result in the evolution of the perfect organism. A 'good enough' mutation will achieve dominance if it happens in the right place at the right time, because of the sensitivity of the evolutionary process to initial conditions: that is, an initial slim advantage may translate into a prolonged period of dominance, without necessarily being optimal".[296]

He could equally have been describing the rapid spread and establishment of early Christianity and Islam, or Mormonism. After all, following its adoption by the Roman empire, Christianity replaced polytheism in Europe for much the same reasons that Latin became Europe's *lingua franca*. A similar ability to 'outlast' their initial benefits may explain why placebo effects can be very persistent.

A medically important aspect of any attempt to describe and understand these extreme religious experiences is that some of the most celebrated religious founders and figures may have had the condition called psychomotor or temporal lobe epilepsy (TLE) that I briefly mentioned in Chapter 11. TLE is the archetypal 'brainstorm' and while in most cases, both the abnormal behaviour and the disturbances of thought and feeling are short-lived and trivial, they can sometimes be dramatic, as with my double homicide patient,[297] and may also be prolonged. TLE often co-exists with ordinary epileptic seizures but can cause delusions, hallucinations and spectacular disturbances of behaviour without visible convulsions.

Religious delusions are common in all psychotic illnesses. They were even commoner when religion was a more salient feature of daily life but TLE is regularly associated with a syndrome consisting of profound religious or quasi-religious experiences and 'fevers', a tendency to write about them at great length ('graphomania') and the apparent absence of a sense of humour. That accurately describes some of history's most prominent religious figures, from St Paul onwards and the condition is sufficiently well-established to have its own name – the Gastaut-Geschwind syndrome. Despite the caveats that apply to all retrospective and historical diagnosis, there is persuasive evidence that this syndrome has helped to change the course of history. Bear in mind that epilepsy is usually one of the more obvious and distinct diagnoses and its main features are easily recognisable from descriptions written many centuries before the time of Hippocrates. In its common and classic form, epilepsy is much easier to diagnose retrospectively with some confidence than, say, heart or bowel disease, cancer, skin disorders or ordinary fevers.

Brain damage is one of the commonest identifiable causes of epilepsy and in an age when malnutrition was endemic (including malnutrition during pregnancy), when childbirth itself was a perilous business for both mother and baby and when severe illness in infancy and childhood was common, as it still is in many countries, brain damage in early life – and thus epilepsy – occurred much more frequently than it does in prosperous countries today. There were also no effective treatments for it (though an eminent Victorian physician, appropriately surnamed Locock, believed that epilepsy was among the many diseases caused by masturbation. He advised treatment with potassium bromide, a toxic sedative that was supposed to suppress this disgusting and un-British habit.) Furthermore, untreated epilepsy often gets worse because repeated seizures can cause further brain damage.

In a religion-obsessed age, the strange feelings, sometimes amounting to vivid auditory and visual hallucinations, that some epileptics experience before or during a seizure (the 'aura') were interpreted in religious terms, as were the delusions and hallucinations of schizophrenia. It is probable that most of the visible convulsions of religious ecstasy had a purely psychological and cultural origin, like those of the *convulsionnaires* of St. Médard. Some important religious figures, however, are widely believed by neurologists[298] to have suffered from TLE. They include Mohammed, Joan of Arc and St Teresa of Avila and later ones such as Joseph Smith, the founder of Mormonism. A rare dissenting paper, by a Muslim physician possibly fearful of the personal and professional consequences of endorsing such *lèse majesté*, absolves Mohammed.[299]

Among Haitians, Voodoo is the main religion and like the related syncretic religions in Brazil, Cuba and other Caribbean islands, it is "not substantially different from the Dahomean cults of the 17th and 18th century, except for human sacrifice, which was then widely practised. ...Worship and possessions by spirits *(loas)* are [its] essence" and its adherents "voluntarily place themselves under the authority of some priest/priestess." However, neurologists in nearby Miami described five patients from the Haitian diaspora in whom various types of epilepsy, including TLE, "were attributed to possession by Voodoo spirits". In one case, a prolonged and difficult birth that modern obstetrics would have avoided was the probable cause of the underlying brain damage. In another, the priest attributed his failure to exorcise "*l'envois morts*... a feared Voodoo curse" to "the strong hold of the spirit". All improved considerably with anti-epileptic medication.[300] Profound mystical experiences happen to ordinary, non-epileptic people but monotheists tend to see them as confirming religious dogmas whereas members of Eastern religions (and atheists) are more likely to describe them in terms of oneness with the universe.[301]

Hallucinogenic drugs have been used by shamans in healing ceremonies for thousands of years and their modern descendants in

Mexico, Brazil, Gabon and elsewhere still use them. Sometimes, both shaman and patient take the drugs as a way of communicating with the tribal gods. In other cultures, only the shaman takes them. Some plant extracts can induce epileptic fits, like the camphor that was used to induce therapeutic seizures before electrically-induced convulsions made it redundant. They might have been used to induce 'feverish', William James varieties of epileptic seizure. The hallucinatory effects of TLE might also have been spontaneously exploited for healing ceremonies by shamans. In people predisposed to epilepsy, deliberate or unwitting over-breathing for as little as two minutes can provoke seizure activity in the temporal lobes and more generally.

The retrospective diagnoses of TLE are often based on apparently first-hand accounts from contemporary observers but St Paul's own account of his dramatic conversion, if authentic, is also suggestive of TLE. The list of well-documented and highly probable later sufferers whose religious beliefs were both strong and influential includes Emanuel Swedenborg, St Teresa of Lisieux and Fyodor Dostoyevsky. Prof. Michael Trimble has also examined the evidence that poetical, musical and religious fervour (and talent) involve similar brain areas and that the right temporal lobe may be particularly important.

Even with modern diagnostic techniques, the diagnosis can be difficult because sometimes 'real' convulsions – the kind that are always accompanied by characteristic changes in brain electrical activity, detectable on the electro-encephalogram (EEG) – can coexist in the same patient with pseudo-convulsions of the psychogenic, psycho-cultural, *convulsionnaire* or 'hysterical' kind. To make matters even more complicated, the same brain damage that can cause genuine epilepsy may also make individuals more susceptible to the types of abnormal behaviour that we label psychogenic or hysterical.

Such patients can present complex diagnostic challenges in modern neuropsychiatry that may only be resolved by simultaneous 24-hour EEG and video monitoring to see whether the apparent seizures coincide precisely with characteristic changes in the brain's electrical activity. Conversely, by stimulating specific brain areas with strong external magnetic fields, people can be made to experience sensations that are often described as, in some sense, 'spiritual'. The commonest kind involves a 'sensed presence' or an 'out of body' experience and in religious people, these sensations are usually described in religious terms and ascribed to divine power. Non-religious people "attribute the phenomena to their own cognitive processes".[302] Not everyone experiences these strange sensations during electromagnetic stimulation and Richard Dawkins is said to have been one of the non-responders. According to taste, his detractors or admirers will presumably see that as showing either a deplorable insensitivity to the reality of God's power or that he is the fortunate owner of a brain that is less easily misled than other brains by minor variations in neurophysiological activity. I haven't tried it myself but a researcher did once apply a more powerful magnetic field over the part of my brain that controls movement. It caused my left arm to rise without conscious effort and was certainly a strange and very impressive experience.

Finally, in an age and a country where most citizens, especially indigenous ones, no longer regard religion as an important part of their life or their identity, we need to remind ourselves that things used to be very different. Barely a century ago in some parts of Britain, religious revivals "centred on travelling preachers, who called the faithful to testify to being 'chosen' by public demonstrations of belief, generated intense experiences and enthusiasm". Similar revivals, sometimes called 'Great Awakenings' had occurred in both Britain and its North American colonies before and after Independence from the 18th to the mid-19th century and beyond. In North Wales during one such revival in 1904-5, the county asylum at Denbigh admitted a small but steady flow of patients with acute and severe psychotic reactions.[303] They had not just been briefly overcome or elated by religious enthusiasm or exhaustion and only needed a few days of rest and some sleeping tablets. These casualties of 'religious fever' stayed in hospital for an average of 225 days, though they were discharged much more quickly than patients with schizophrenia who, in an age that lacked effective anti-psychotic drugs, stayed for over ten years on average. Also unlike patients with schizophrenia or severe bipolar illness, they nearly all needed only that single admission throughout their lives. In 1905, the peak year, these acute religious psychoses accounted for a significant increase in admissions and they outnumbered the similar acute psychoses that were caused by different forms of severe psychological or physiological stress, notably the 'puerperal' psychosis that still follows about one in every thousand full-term childbirths. (The incidence of psychosis after abortion is five times *lower*.)[304] Another interesting feature of the psychoses was that they were significantly commoner in men aged 15-35 than in any other group of either sex. There is no further breakdown of this group by age but adolescents may well have been particularly over-represented, for adolescence is often a time of strong religious feelings, combined with a brain that is still developing. A former bishop of Birmingham, Hugh Montefiore, born into a prominent Jewish family, had a vision of Jesus and converted to Christianity while still a schoolboy.

My reason for mentioning this bit of relatively recent history is not to blame religion for making a few people psychotic. It is to note again that regardless of the god that is worshipped or the specific beliefs of a particular religion or sect, some of the procedures that are common to nearly all religions and used to be practised more frequently here, can have very profound effects on the human mind and human behaviour. It is another reason why we should not be surprised at the power of placebo, nocebo and non-specific effects that involve similar mechanisms of suggestion, arousal, charisma, expectation, hope and fear.

Chapter 20
The misdiagnosis of King George III
Whatever happened to the blue urine?

Thanks to Alan Bennett (whom God preserve) almost everyone knows that poor old Mad King George wasn't really mad at all. Thanks to Alan Bennett, almost everyone is mistaken about this but let's not spoil a good story; not yet, anyway. This chapter uses a particularly famous case-history to show how easy it is for both doctors and their patients to believe that any improvement that follows a particular intervention must be due to the treatment and not simply a fluctuation in the natural, untreated course of the disease. For several centuries, philosophers have called this logical error, exemplified by the elephant joke, *post hoc, ergo propter hoc.* (After X, therefore because of X.)

The theory that 'Farmer George' had a rare metabolic disorder called porphyria and not 'real' insanity didn't originate with Bennett. Just as I was beginning my psychiatric training, the paper that started this little diagnostic, philosophical and theatrical cottage industry appeared in the *British Medical Journal*[305] and was widely discussed by trainees and trainers alike. Most of my teachers were not impressed by the argument that madness due to porphyria was somehow very different from madness due to – well, whatever 'ordinary' madness was due to. (We still haven't really found out.) They also muttered, rather unkindly, that the authors of the paper, Drs Richard Hunter and Ida Macalpine, were an unhealthily close mother-and-son dyad and thus perhaps Not Quite Sound. As we'll see, my teachers were broadly correct on this point but not for the reasons they gave us at the time. In any case, the few national and international experts on porphyria soon weighed in, claiming that the psychiatric disturbances that occasionally – but by no means invariably – accompanied porphyria weren't at all like those that characterised King George's mental illness. Several other features also made the diagnosis very doubtful. Still, one had to admire Hunter and Macalpine's nerve and persistence in asking the British and continental descendants of the Hanoverian dynasty, many still living in their palaces and schlosses, for specimens of royal wee and ducal turds to analyse for their porphyrin content.[306] In a few cases, they reported, cooperation was not forthcoming.

On one point there is no disagreement. For varying periods, George III was so disturbed, divorced from reality and incapable of sensible discussion that he was unable to do his rather important job; and not just a little bit unable but absolutely, totally unable. His problems were not that he was too weak, feverish, breathless or doubled up with pain to meet his ministers or sign documents and neither had he suffered a stroke that affected his speech. In other words, they were not physical problems, so they must have been broadly behavioural or psychiatric problems, and serious ones at that. In short, he was mentally ill or – in the vernacular of his time and of ours – mad. It is true that temporary mental disturbance following, say, a head injury, a very bad LSD trip or extreme psychological or emotional stress, may not be regarded as 'ordinary' insanity even if it is very severe, provided that it really is temporary and, even more important, doesn't recur, but none of these mitigating factors applied to King George. In any case, even if he had become deranged for long periods after a severe head injury or, as sometimes happens, as part of an underlying epileptic disorder, he would still have been called Mad King George and Britain would still have experienced the same constitutional and political consequences. Finally, if one of the things that worries people about 'ordinary' madness is that it sometimes runs in families, then porphyria – a classic genetic disorder – is surely just as worrying in that respect as schizophrenia or manic-depressive illness.

Bennett – one of my favourite modern comic dramatists, by the way – shouldn't perhaps be blamed too much for taking up the Hunter and Macalpine theory. He is, it's true, an Oxford history graduate (with first class honours) and subsequently taught the subject there for a while but he has made his living as a playwright, not a historian and at least he didn't dramatise a completely imaginary murder plot involving Mozart and Salieri, as Peter Schaffer did with *Amadeus* (and as Pushkin and Rimsky-Korsakov did before Schaffer[307]). We live in an age that is not merely undeferential but positively anti-deferential and whatever the cause of the King's madness, the play gave lots of scope for ridiculing the activities of his medical attendants, with perhaps some implications that care of the mentally ill is still not one of modern medicine's bigger triumphs. The medical story hinges on the failure of the mad-doctors to notice that the royal urine had turned blue, though it is not suggested that they ought to have known about porphyria, which wasn't described until the late 19th century. (Neither was the ultra-violet light that makes diagnosing porphyria easy if it happens to illuminate your urine stream, thus making it fluoresce in a darkened room.)

History is rather more prone to error and bias than science, and historical diagnosis is no exception. Repeatability and predictability are crucial aspects of science. History, by definition, is unrepeatable and unpredictable and can only be reconstructed from the available evidence. (As Samuel Butler quipped: "Though God cannot alter the past, historians can: it is perhaps because they can be useful to Him in this respect that He tolerates their existence.") New evidence – or a more diligent and less partisan examination of old evidence - can mean new history and this is what has happened with the porphyria theory. Another pair of researchers, Peters and Wilkinson, have re-examined the porphyria hypothesis and the documentary evidence relied on by Hunter and Macalpine.[308] This pair are, as far as I know, unrelated and neither of them is a psychiatrist but Wilkinson is a historian and Peters is a retired British professor of medicine who, rather unusually, has substantial clinical experience of the various types of porphyria. What they have discovered is an object lesson in how a micro-ideology can completely distort the assessment of evidence. In particular, they have shown that the 'blue urine' story, so crucial to the impact of Bennett's play and subsequent film, is unsupported even by the documents cited by Hunter and Macalpine, who gave it an importance that it does not deserve.

In addition to re-examining the documents that were available to Hunter and Macalpine, they also looked at the Hunter-Macalpine notes and correspondence, now in the Cambridge University Library, which gave some disturbing insights into the way mother and son had worked:

> "Macalpine and Hunter ... were driven by deep convictions about the nature of mental illness, to research the 'madness' of George III. They ... believed that mental illnesses were primarily caused by physical diseases, most of which were still waiting to be discovered. [and] were therefore psychologically predisposed to favour a diagnosis of porphyria because it supported their personal agenda: 'the royal malady may perhaps – as in 1788 – serve psychiatry by indicating the direction of its future progress'."

These 'deep convictions' made them ignore two very important flaws in their argument. Firstly, given that the King's episodes of illness lasted for months or even years at a time and were supposedly characterised by blue urine *throughout the period of his illness*, it is bizarre that Hunter and MacAlpine ignored the detailed daily reports on the royal urine showing it to be entirely normal in colour. (In those technology-lite days, daily descriptions of stools and urine were the equivalent of today's daily temperature and blood-pressure charts and electrocardiographic monitoring.) Secondly, if the urine in porphyria has an abnormal colour, that colour is 'a dark reddish-brown'. Apart from a brief episode late in his life, which clearly refers to blood in the urine (probably from a bladder stone) no such reddish-brown colour was reported. Thirdly – and most damning of all – there is only one alleged reference to 'bluish' urine in the hand-written contemporary notes but Peters and Wilkinson conclude from both the manuscript and the context that the word in question is 'between', not 'bluish'. This literal misreading of history refers, in any case, not to the colour of the urine but to the timing of some medication. There is no mention of urine at all in the relevant extracts from the original papers.

Finally, Peters and Wilkinson found that in the days before a single, isolated report of urine that 'left a pale blue ring on the glass near the upper surface' (but was not described as uniformly blue in colour) the King had been given medicine containing gentian (the extract of a plant that produces a dark blue-violet dye as well as having a bitter taste that was thought to aid digestion) which suggests an alternative explanation. Yet the film version in particular stresses the alleged return of normal colour in the urine when the King suddenly recovers enough to go to Parliament and thwart the takeover plans of his dissolute son, the future George IV. "Piss the elder," says one of the attendants "and piss the younger", making a pun on the name of the Prime Minister, William Pitt the Younger before throwing both specimens away. The old, unhealthy urine, we are expected to believe, is blue. The new, healthy specimen is not. Ironically, although Hunter and Macalpine hoped that their line of enquiry might lead to improvements in the care of psychiatric patients, Peters notes that following the publication of their papers and the subsequent increased concern that psychiatrists might be missing cases of porphyria, "some 15,000 patients in south-west London were screened for porphyria without a single case being identified. Surely the money involved could have been better used to improve patient care?"[309]

The most likely psychiatric diagnosis – and the one favoured by most psycho-historians as well as by my teachers in the mid 1960s – is the predominantly manic form of manic-depressive psychosis (or 'bipolar I disorder' as it is usually called now) with the later development of Alzheimer or multi-infarct dementia (i.e. dementia caused by multiple mini-strokes). The later onset of dementia is strongly supported by the characteristic deterioration in the King's handwriting and signature that has been shown to correlate well with the neuropsychological changes in dementia. Recurrent mania is also consistent with the George's rapid and continuous speech and his tendency to flit from one topic to another even when well - the subjects of several satirical poems. While most bipolar patients have both manic and depressed episodes, some have predominantly one or the other and like most psychiatrists, I have seen a few 'pure' recurrent manic patients. Today, manic-depressive illness often responds well to treatment. RCTs show that lithium and other drugs reduce the frequency, severity and length of episodes compared with placebo medication and, of course, the usual nursing and psychological interventions that both placebo and 'active' patients received as well.[310] The fact that lithium and other mood-stabilising drugs can significantly increase the length of remissions between episodes indicates that they have an effect – however poorly-understood – on the basic disease process, whatever it is. If they gave only symptomatic relief as with opiates for pain, we might expect them to reduce the severity but not the duration or frequency of episodes.

Before the lithium era, which coincided with the introduction of other drugs that had useful rather than spectacular effects on schizophrenia and depression compared with placebo, manic-depressive patients often had episodes of mania or depression that lasted for months or years. Some of them were so depressed and inert that they did not eat and died in hospital from malnourishment or from infections made worse by their weakened condition. Some manic patients may have died from heart disease aggravated by excessive activity and George III, who was not exactly slender in later life, may have been lucky in this respect at least. However, several of his episodes were relatively short and, as we would now say, self-limiting. As previously noted, when you are treating someone, your treatment tends to get – and certainly to take – the credit when things go well. And until the arrival of the compensation culture a few decades ago, if things went badly, well, that's just the way things were. Barring major negligence, nobody - including God - was to blame. That was especially the case if the patient survived, even if he remained ill, as with George III. His 'specialist' or 'mad doctor', the Rev. Dr Francis Willis, had to put up with some criticism, especially from rival doctors, but the fact that the king enjoyed several long remissions was seen as vindicating his methods. However, he failed to do as well with the Queen of Portugal – Maria the Pious or, more unkindly, Maria the Mad – who became insane in her 50s and stayed that way, though his role was only advisory and her actual treatment was in the hands of Portuguese doctors. The memorial in his local church claims that Willis, who lived to be 90, was 'happily the chief agent in removing the malady which affected his present majesty in the year 1789'. In reality, the most likely explanation is that, as Voltaire noted of doctors generally, being a good physician in Georgian Britain simply meant amusing the patient while

Nature cured him – or didn't, as was often the case. It still is the case, even if we can keep that unhelpful part of Nature at bay for rather longer these days. Dr Willis's treatment almost certainly had no effect on the course or severity of his royal patient's illness.

As we have seen, an earlier monarch, Elizabeth's successor James I of England and VI of Scotland, had a more sceptical view of such *post hoc* therapeutic claims and expressed it in language that is colourful but surprisingly scientific and still very readable. King James was one of the earliest anti-smoking campaigners and he criticised it not just because, like me, he regarded smoking as a messy, malodorous and antisocial habit as well as an unhealthy one ('...lothsome to the eye, hatefull to the Nose, harmefull to the braine, dangerous to the Lungs, and in the blacke stinking fume thereof, neerest resembling the horrible Stigian smoke of the pit that is bottomelesse.') but also because many of those who used and sold the fashionable new import claimed that it actually cured several diseases. If the *Daily Mail* had existed then, it would surely have promoted tobacco on its health pages but James demolished the *post hoc, ergo propter hoc* arguments on which many therapeutic claims were based (and still are in much of Complementary and Alternative Medicine):

Good old James. It would be difficult to find a better description from Early Modern Europe, especially "the apprehension and conceit of the patient hath by wakening and uniting the vitall spirits, and so strengthening nature, a great power and vertue, to cure divers diseases.", of the placebo effect in both patient and doctor, of spontaneous recovery and of what was still called, in my student days, the *vis medicatrix naturae* – the healing power of (unassisted) nature.

There's an interesting separate diagnostic debate about King James. Not content with misdiagnosing George III, Hunter and Macalpine claimed that several of George's ancestors had porphyria, including James and his son Prince Henry, who died in his teens. Peters and his colleagues show that there is no evidence for the claim but when they fed the numerous contemporary medical and other descriptions of James (including his post-mortem examination) into a diagnostic computer programme normally used for living patients, it surprised them by coming up with an even rarer condition than porphyria, a mild version of Lesch-Nyhan syndrome. This condition was only described in the 1960s and the milder forms were recognised even more recently. One of its features is very high uric acid levels, leading to gout. James was certainly gouty and one of his kidneys was badly damaged by stones that were probably due to the same cause.[311] The kidney disease, in turn, probably caused the high blood pressure that would explain both his enlarged heart and the stroke that killed him.

Of course, the fun thing about historical diagnosis is that in most cases, nobody can ever be categorically proved right or wrong. Poor old Farmer George *might* have had some kind of porphyria, even if it never turned his urine the appropriate colour, as Bennett's theatrical and cinematic accounts argue that it did, but that's not the same as proving that porphyria *caused* his insanity. You would expect an inheritable disorder like porphyria to be more common in a family where intermarriage was built into the system. We know how Queen Victoria spread haemophilia through half the monarchies of Europe through a genetic mutation that evidently first appeared in her father. However if one of her haemophilic descendants had also been mentally ill, we wouldn't have said the insanity was really due to haemophilia. We would have said it was a predictable coincidence, because haemophilia of itself is not associated with insanity. And neither, as a rule, are the porphyrias.

Chapter 21
Suicide prevention and the Samaritans
Misplaced therapeutic optimism and mission creep

The Samaritans was founded by a Church of England vicar, the Reverend (later Prebendary) Chad Varah. It was never a sectarian or even a religious organization but it originated in a pastoral experience that must still be familiar to parish priests and must have been even more familiar when the church played a bigger part in most people's lives. A 14-year-old country girl, misinterpreting her first menstrual periods as a sign of sexually transmitted disease, killed herself; Varah had to conduct her funeral service. That was in the 1930s when adolescent ignorance about sexual matters was much commoner than it is today.

After the war, Varah moved to London where, as well as getting involved in sex education, he set up the Samaritans in 1953 with the very specific purpose of 'befriend[ing] the suicidal and despairing'. Who could possibly complain? That sort of thing was surely one of the traditional roles of the clergy, especially when attempting suicide was a felony (derived from Canon Law) that was still regularly prosecuted and sometimes punished by imprisonment right up to its decriminalization in 1961. What sort of person, however cynical, would even demand evidence that the Samaritans actually had any useful effect on the suicide rate? The Samaritans were trying to help and were a volunteer organization making no demands on the public purse.

The effectiveness of the Samaritans would probably not have been questioned, even by any of the usual academic suspects, had not a sociologist, Christopher Bagley, produced a paper in the late 1960s claiming to show that the geographical growth of the Samaritans since their foundation had been paralleled by a fall in suicide in those areas where Samaritans branches existed but not in areas where they had not yet been established.[312] Bear in mind that during the period covered by Bagley's research, making a phone call outside your local area was neither easy nor cheap and many callers would have had to use public telephone boxes. I don't recall whether this claim was accompanied by suggestions that the Samaritans should therefore receive public money for training and administrative expenses but it would hardly have been surprising. The late 1960s were a time of both social ferment and optimism and a recently re-elected Labour government might well have been sympathetic to the idea. The Samaritans have certainly received modest subsidies from the government in recent years.

I was doing my psychiatric training when Bagley's study appeared and it caused a lot of interest. His claim seemed intrinsically plausible and I don't recall that any of us took against it on ideological grounds. Suicidal overdosers arriving in Casualty represented most of our emergency work and it was obvious that many of them had understandable reasons for feeling unhappy. Often they had few suitable friends and family members with whom they might share their problems and thus perhaps reduce them. By the late 1970s, overdoses, usually but not always with some suicidal intent, had become the commonest reason for admission to acute female medical wards. It was even predicted,[313] incorrectly, as it turned out,[314] that at current rates of increase, every acute female medical bed in Britain would be filled with an overdose patient by 1984.

Unfortunately for Bagley and the Samaritans, the study had two big flaws. One was in its method of statistical analysis, as shown in subsequent publications[315] – and as eventually more-or-less accepted by Bagley himself, to do him credit. It was a few years before the study could be replicated using data that had accumulated after 1968 and during that time, belief in the 'Samaritan Effect' might have been maintained but for one curious feature of Bagley's findings. During the sixties, suicide rates for the traditional British method since about 1920, putting your head in an unlit gas oven, really had fallen but the rates for other methods had either stayed the same or, especially for self-poisoning with tablets, increased. If the 'Samaritan Effect' existed, it seemingly influenced only those who intended to use gas ovens for suicide and not those choosing other methods, which was on the face of it unlikely.

The explanation was not the sympathetic attitudes and conversations of the mainly middle-class and often female Samaritan volunteers but the efforts of a more uncouth group consisting exclusively of men with blue collars and bluer language who had drilled holes in the bed of the North Sea, thus enabling the replacement of poisonous coal-gas, rich in carbon monoxide, with non-toxic natural gas. Nobody seems to have predicted the change in suicide rates that this would cause but British rates fell steadily from a post-war peak in 1963, when natural gas was introduced, until 1975, when with the exception of Northern Ireland, every town in the realm had been converted to natural gas.

Bagley did not surrender immediately. He and his defenders pointed out that while natural gas had been introduced at the same time in several other countries bordering the North Sea, only in Britain had the suicide rate fallen significantly and only in Britain had the Samaritans, or anything like them in terms of a country-wide service, come into existence. The explanation turned out to be a socio-economic one. Britain, the pioneer of the industrial revolution and for long its most urbanized manifestation, was the first country in Europe to have a national network of coal-gas supplies, which reached many houses towards the end of the 19th century. The 1890s saw the introduction and mass-production of gas cookers that soon replaced the dirty and labour-intensive coal- or wood-burning kitchen ranges on which most households had cooked for the previous century or so.

Nobody seems to have studied how it came about but by the 1920s, the knowledge that gas ovens were a fairly reliable way of ending it all had reached most of Britain. From that time, coal-gas poisoning overtook all the more traditional methods of suicide – hanging, drowning, stabbing or nasty poisons like arsenic, bleach or strychnine that were the ones mainly used before sleeping pills became available in the late 19th century. Jumping from a height was not easy when most people lived in one- or two-storey homes. Opium, though reasonably lethal in overdose, widely consumed and obtainable without prescription until 1916, never became popular as a method of suicide and unlike many European countries, 20th century Britain had relatively few gun-owners. Other North Sea-facing countries did not develop coal-gas supplies to the same extent and at the same time. For that and other reasons, coal-gas suicide never became as common as it was in Britain. Other methods predominated and consequently, the introduction of natural gas in those countries had a much smaller effect on national suicide rates.

Varah continued to have a senior role and was its president until 1986 but gradually became disenchanted with it. Like many organisations established to supply a particular need, the Samaritans became a classic example of 'mission creep' until Stonewall took the crown. When he finally broke with them in 2004, Varah complained that the service he had established in the hope of helping suicidal or similarly desperate people had now become just a source of 'emotional support' in general. Ironically, the Samaritans provide a service not only for those who use its telephone lines but also for those who take the calls. Getting involved in the business of helping one's fellow-human beings can be a deeply satisfying and mood-enhancing experience, as most doctors will quickly confirm, at least in their younger and more enthusiastic days. For both helper and helped, this satisfaction often persists even when the help provided is not objectively helpful.

But surely, most people might argue, there is a need for that kind of well-intentioned effort in our fractured society in which the support of the traditional nuclear and extended family is increasingly hard to find? They may be right but several decades ago, I described what the medical journalist and writer Theodore Dalrymple was kind enough to call 'Brewer's Law'. Like Parkinson's Law, which inspired the analogy ('work expands so as to occupy the time available for its completion') Brewer's Law states that 'unhappiness increases so as to occupy the facilities for its relief'. We live in a time of unprecedented access to sources of help and support that are not far removed from what the Samaritans in their new incarnation now provide. We also live in a time where the number of people suffering from what are classed as psychiatric or 'mental health' conditions, many of them receiving short- or long-term sickness benefit, has increased, is increasing and shows little sign of diminishing. It has been argued that these trends might, just possibly, be causally related because people may undervalue their own resilience and thus perceive themselves as more dependent on external assistance than might otherwise have been the case.

It would be difficult to conduct a controlled study to resolve this argument but hints are to be had from two sources, one a planned study and the other an unplanned, non-randomised 'natural experiment' that has been so often repeated that the results are hard to ignore. The planned study was published in 1978[316] and examined the effect of an 'intensive' social work intervention, vs the standard non-intensive one with much less input by social workers, on the incidence of suicide attempts in a group of London general practice patients who had already made one such attempt. All research shows, unsurprisingly, that people who have made a suicide attempt are much more likely to make future attempts than people who have never attempted suicide. Around 20% of them typically make a further attempt within a year, so it made both clinical and economic sense to concentrate preventive interventions on a group who had very clearly demonstrated their vulnerability. Suicide is a major cause of death among young people in industrialised societies (several agrarian ones too, notably Sri Lanka and rural China) now that they rarely die from infectious diseases. Most of those who attempt suicide do not go on to kill themselves but quite a few do. Showing that intensive social work was effective would help to plan appropriate services for reducing a particularly tragic cause of death, especially for young suicides who might have learned better survival skills if they hadn't died before they had a chance to acquire them. It might also provide a better understanding of the reasons why people kill themselves.

Alas, there was no difference between the 'intensive' and standard groups in the incidence of further attempts. You might have thought that would be the end of the matter, especially if previous and subsequent attempts at suicide prevention with such techniques proved equally disappointing or only marginal, as has generally been the case. You would have been wrong. Searching desperately for some justification for their efforts, and perhaps for their existence as an independent profession, the social worker authors seized on a tiny silver lining to the annoying cloud of reality that had emerged from their study. They might have been less annoyed if they had been familiar with the null hypothesis.

Significantly more 'intensive' than control patients reported that they had received 'a lot of help' or that they were 'very satisfied with the service'. 'Intensive' patients also reported significant differences, evidently regarded by the authors as useful or desirable, in the way that they perceived certain social problems. On these slender grounds, the authors tried to justify the use of the more intensive and thus more expensive social work intervention but the patients received this intervention because – and only because – they had taken an overdose. They did not receive it in order to change the way they viewed certain social problems. In any case, even if it did change their views, the changes didn't make them any happier, since there was no difference between the groups on a rating scale for depression four months after the initial overdose. Like these social workers, researchers in controlled trials of drugs quite often seize on minor incidental findings that were not among the original aims of the study and may not have any significant clinical benefit.

It is possible that something similar happens as a result of Samaritan activities; that is, people may feel better for making contact without necessarily functioning better. Alternatively, improvements in feeling and/or function may be a non-specific effect of human contact. None of this is an argument for abolishing the Samaritans and similar considerations and reservations apply to many forms of counselling and psychotherapy. It is, though, an argument for therapeutic modesty when it comes to claims that if the Samaritans did not exist, the sum of human happiness would be greatly reduced. It is also a reason for wondering whether there can be such a thing as too much counselling and 'therapy'.

The 'natural experiment' takes place every time a country goes to war with another country. (Civil wars may be a different matter). Without exception, this sort of war causes the suicide rate to plummet, except right at the end, when there may be a flurry of suicides among the defeated for reasons of military honour, defiance or fear of vengeance by the victors, as happened in both Germany and Japan in 1945. When WW2 began, tens of thousands of emergency psychiatric beds were hurriedly planned for the massive psychiatric casualties that everyone expected to follow the bombing of our cities. Not one of them was needed. The suicide rate declined consistently by about a third between 1938 and 1944. War makes most survivors more resilient, not less, whether they live in London, Berlin, Aleppo, Leningrad or Gaza.

The national suicide statistics tell us only about deaths from suicide that took place within Britain and exclude suicides among the armed forces in the various theatres of war. It's a fascinating and largely unexplored area, though well outside the scope of this chapter but an epidemiologist I know who tried to explore it recalled a discussion with an elderly desk-warrior in the Ministry of Defence. The warrior told him that quite a few exhausted and demoralized British soldiers effectively committed suicide during WW2 by single-handedly charging the enemy lines, so that the enemy would save them the trouble and shame of shooting themselves. Whether or not they survived, they were usually given a medal so as not to damage morale but sometimes, the enemy were even more exhausted and demoralised than the lone, suicidal British soldier and unexpectedly surrendered to him.

Chapter 22
Candide and the doctors

Dr. Matthew Turner of Liverpool, Britain's first atheist to go public

Ubi tres physici, ibi duo athei. (Where there are three doctors, there you will find two atheists.)
Mediaeval saying, attribution unknown.
That society which suffers by truth should be otherwise constituted.
Dr Matthew Turner.

Daily and intimate clinical exposure to unpleasant aspects of life that the unmedical see only occasionally, if at all, may be one reason why doctors were prominent among early atheists. Never send to know for whom the bell tolls? Medical students learned sooner than most of their contemporaries that it tolled for them as well as for their patients. More than other students, they learned just how random, unpleasant, unfair and dangerous the world can be and thus how questionable is the idea of a benevolent deity in charge of the whole precarious business. A realisation that apparently struck Voltaire only when he was 60, after news of the 1755 Lisbon earthquake, fire and tsunami reached Europe's cities, inspiring him to write *Candide,* may hit medical students the moment they enter the hospital wards in their late teens or early twenties, if it has not occurred to them earlier.

One of the first patients I saw as a student was a paraplegic teenager with severe spina bifida and a fluid-filled sac the size of a football over the base of his spine. This made it impossible for him to lie on his back or side and he had been nursed face-downwards for all of his 16 years with no control of his bladder and bowels. He was old enough, intelligent enough and adolescent enough to know what he was missing and this knowledge had not made him happy. Those physical, psychological and spiritual burdens would have been a challenge for anyone but Fate was not satisfied. He developed a cancer in the tissues of the sac that filled the end of his short and miserable existence with even more pain and indignity. Soon after qualifying as a doctor, the poet John Keats, wrote "While we are laughing, the seed of some trouble is put into the wide arable land of events – while we are laughing, it sprouts, it grows and suddenly bears a poison fruit which we must pluck."[317] Within two years, Keats himself had plucked the poison fruit of tuberculosis and died aged only tenty-five. Plenty of people abandon their religious beliefs without seeing this sort of thing, but it helps.

It is possible to ignore the suffering of patients or treat it as essentially normal and, up to a point, unavoidable. We soon learn not to cry in front of our patients and from there it is an easy step to not crying at all; and also to not thinking very much about the Problem of Suffering. The more sensitive among us may move to areas of medicine that involve little personal contact with real, living (and dying) patients – public health, health education and health politics, for example. If we choose family planning, school health or sports medicine, we shall see relatively few patients who confront us with spiritually troubling illnesses. For doctors in ordinary medical practice who find it difficult to ignore or evade The Problem, there are two options. Those who believe in a god have somehow to square the existence of suffering with divine benevolence. (God moves in mysterious ways; it is part of His plan, even if we cannot see it; suffering is ennobling; it must be due to individual – or original – sin.) If they cannot square this circle of medical reality, they may reach the opposite conclusion – that there is no god (atheism) or that if there is one, he may have created the world but is a mere 'divine shipbuilder'. This god sets his creation afloat but is not subsequently concerned with the fate or suffering of individual passengers (deism).

By mediaeval times, it had become very dangerous to voice heresies, especially radical and fundamental ones such as atheism. The Roman Inquisition successfully eliminated the Cathars in the 13th Century, 200 years before its Spanish franchise set to work. It is hardly surprising that none of the names of those mediaeval multiples of the *duo athei* has come down to us but in 1553, the physician-philosopher Miguel Servetus – possible discoverer, before William Harvey, of the circulation of the blood – was burnt alive in Geneva on the orders of John Calvin just for having doubts about the Trinity.[318] Another prominent physician-philosopher, Pietro Pomponazzi, a teacher at the ancient university and medical school of Padua, somehow got away with denying immortality "about as unequivocally as any man of his day".[319] Long before that, the physician-philosopher Averroes, a product of the Golden Age of science and religious coexistence in Islamic Spain, had reached the same conclusion. The medical and philosophical textbooks written by Averroes were popular in late mediaeval and early Renaissance medical schools and in consequence, "medical men began to be considered freethinkers". We don't know how many other physicians had similar doubts but kept them to themselves for fear of the rack and the flames, or of social and professional ostracism. In any case, it wasn't only doctors who kept their thoughts to themselves. Until well into the 18th Century, *nobody* in Europe published an overtly and uncompromisingly atheist document, apart from Kazimierz Łyszczyński and the village priest Jean Meslier, but as Pierre Bayle, whose sceptical writings Meslier had read, pointed out; "...to be not a theist or [the same thing] an atheist, it is not necessary to affirm that theism is false; it is enough to regard it as a problem".

In Britain, the first doctor known to be *suspected* of atheism was Dr Archibald Pitcairne (1652-1713). Edinburgh's leading physician, he was also famed for his prodigious drinking and his many pamphlets and diatribes against the Presbyterian Church. He was almost certainly an atheist but an Edinburgh student called Thomas Aikenhead was hanged in 1697 for merely voicing atheist thoughts and like Baron d'Holbach, Pitcairne wisely opted for discretion. The first person in Britain known to have broken this silence of the fearful in print without unpleasant consequences was a Liverpool physician, Matthew Turner. We first hear of him when he advertised his services in the *Liverpool Chronicle and Marine Gazetteer* of May 6th 1757:

> 'A Lying-in [i.e. maternity] hospital in this town [many charitably] disposed Persons have desired, and thought very necessary; ... I do hereby inform the Public that I am ready to attend and assist to the best of my power Gratis, all married women, living within the limits of this town, whose Cases in Labour are Difficult or Dangerous, so that the mid-wife is at a loss, or unable alone to perform her Office, provided they are not able to pay.

After mentioning that he had studied at 'two of the Chief Schools of that Art in Europe', he added:

> NB. 'Tis hoped that the Gentlewomen who practise Midwifery in town, will not look upon anything here mentioned as designed to prejudice or undervalue them: the design being only to give them assistance when 'tis wanted, which I Judge may be offered to them in the manner here proposed, without any Impeachment of their abilities, by those who may be allowed to have had better Opportunities of acquiring skill in the Profession than the Practitioners of Their Sex usually have.'[320]

Turner was very progressive by the standards of the time, though Liverpool, a major slaving port, had plenty of God-fearing reactionaries. One anti-slavery pamphlet "led to a Jesuit response from the Rev. Raymond Harris:

> 'Scriptural researches on the Licitness of the Slave Trade, showing its conformity with principles of natural and revealed religion, delineated in the sacred writing of the Word of God'."[321]

Turner was known to associate with other Liverpool freethinkers but he waited until 1781 before committing himself to print. Even then, he sheltered behind his brave publisher, William Hammon but it is almost certain that Turner was the author of *Answer to Dr. Priestley's letters to a philosophical unbeliever.*[322] The Dr Priestley in question was Joseph Priestley, clergyman, early chemist, Fellow of the Royal Society and discoverer of oxygen. A tolerant man, his 1780 *Letters to a philosophical unbeliever* did not suggest that atheists should be punished, only that they were misguided. The fact that Priestly felt it necessary to write the book indicates that the expression of 'unbelief' in various forms was no longer very rare, even if it had not reached the printed page.

Turner mentions Vanini's horrible execution but despite his obvious fears – "he hopes he shall not himself be marked out as an object of persecution." – he did not equivocate. After noting that "No tyranny is greater than that of ecclesiastics. These chain down our very ideas, other tyrants only confine our limbs." and "There are few or none who will venture openly to acknowledge themselves to be atheists.", he marched boldly out of the closet:

> "But as to the question whether there is such an existent Being as an atheist, to put that out of all manner of doubt, I do declare upon my honour that I am one. Be it therefore for the future remembered, that in London in the kingdom of England, in the year of our Lord one thousand seven hundred and eighty-one, a man has publickly declared himself an atheist."

He added that "[a] society which suffers by truth should be otherwise constituted".

I can only speculate that Turner's 'unbelief' in a benevolent deity, or any other kind may have been partly fuelled by his exposure to the daily horrors of 18th century medicine and its considerable limitations. What is not speculation is that Joseph Priestley, his believing but tolerant opponent, had an altogether more rose-tinted, Pollyanna-ish, Panglossian view of life. "I do not like to think or speak of anything unpleasant", Priestley once wrote. "I confide [i.e. believe, trust] in a good Providence, and generally look on the bright side of everything".[323]

Turner had already shown that an atheist could be as charitable as any successful Christian physician. But for an accident of history, he might also have been celebrated as the discoverer of ether anaesthesia, nearly a century before Dr John Warren, the first dean of Harvard's medical school, famously proclaimed, in 1846, 'Gentlemen, this is no humbug'. Ether had been synthesised in the 16th century or earlier by mixing sulphuric acid with alcohol but was not produced in any quantity until the 18th. In 1761, Turner published *An Account of the*

Extraordinary Medicinal Fluid called "Aether" and recommended it, by mouth but not by inhalation, as "a remedy for fits, headaches, gout, rheumatism, pains in the stomach, windy disorders, whooping-cough, asthma and deafness". A historian of Liverpool medical life commented: "Possibly the fact that Turner sold ether at two shillings an ounce made his colleagues somewhat sceptical of its alleged properties."[324] Turner greatly overestimated his healing powers, since oral ether would have had no specifically helpful pharmacological effects on any of those conditions. We can salute Dr Matthew Turner for his personal bravery and independence of thought but as a physician, if not as an early obstetrician, he was just as useless and dangerous as any of his contemporaries.

Even after unbelieving doctors like Turner no longer faced imprisonment or worse, for many years it was often better for their standing in the community, and their income, to keep such views to themselves. Where the unbelief involves Islam, it still is. An ex-Muslim clinical psychologist I know told me that he can only talk about it in the company of like-minded people. Even his wife does not know. Perhaps it was because the writer and physician Somerset Maugham had long ceased practising his profession that he felt able to confide to the Writer's Notebook, published late in his life, that: "I'm glad I don't believe in God".

Chapter 23
Conclusions

What can medicine and religion learn from the placebo effect about each other's practices?

The essential unit of medical practice is the occasion when, in the intimacy of the consulting room, or sick room, a person who is ill, or believes himself to be ill, seeks the advice of a doctor whom he trusts. This is a consultation, and all else in the practice of medicine derives from it.

Sir James Spence. The purpose and practice of medicine.

1: Medicine

After being ignored by most researchers for the past half century of evidence-based medicine, the study of placebo and non-specific effects for their possible deliberate use in treatment is becoming steadily less unthinkable. A compilation of papers from a conference in Canada examined some of those wider implications of placebo effects that I discussed in previous chapters. It barely mentions religion, apart from a sentence on communion wafers in a chapter amusingly headed: 'Placebolicious: the many flavours of placebos in Western diets and food cultures' that is much more erudite than it sounds. It does, though, discuss the theoretical and practical relevance of the concept not just for clinicians but also for ethnologists, medical educators, journalists, politicians, advertisers and – perhaps as a little light relief for the conference delegates – fetishists. As well as the steady stream of research papers from teams led by clinicians like Edzard Ernst and Ted Kaptchuk since the turn of the century and increasing interest in other academic centres, Prof. Fabrizio Benedetti from Turin University, a pioneer of modern placebo research, has put together and updated an encyclopaedia of placebo research that covers the history as well as the possible neurophysiological pathways and psychological processes that mediate placebo phenomena in every area of disease.[325] (He also told me it was about time that somebody wrote about placebo effects in religion.) SIPS – the Society for Interdisciplinary Placebo Studies – is an established and growing organization with well-attended biennial conferences.

It is often claimed that placebo and non-specific effects don't last for long. Apart from the fact that many medical conditions don't last for long either, the claim is untrue. The Duke of Pirajno's serpent-troubled patient seems to have had a lasting recovery. The sham ECT patients are another example. Many RCTs with follow-up periods of as much as a year, including several already discussed, show that improvements in the placebo wing, as compared with no treatment, or a less impressive placebo, or being put on the waiting list after an initial assessment, are often maintained. The pilgrims who leave their wheelchairs and crutches behind at Lourdes and Fatima, like Prof. Ernst's 'spiritually healed' patients who did the same in the more functional ambience of an Exeter NHS clinic, may also remain well or much improved for long periods.

A particularly impressive example of the powerful effects of simply deciding to seek treatment, even if no treatment is actually provided, is one of Britain's few really important contributions to addiction treatment research. The trial of 'Treatment vs Advice' in alcoholism is not as well-known as it should be, possibly because its findings are unwelcome news for expensive residential addiction 'rehabs'. In this 1977 study,[326] married alcohol-abusing men seeking treatment for the first time received a leisurely and lengthy assessment. Married men were chosen so that their wives, who were also interviewed, could provide more independent feedback about their husbands' subsequent drinking and the state of their marriages. Half were randomized to the standard range of treatments, 'best practice' as we would now call it, including advice to attend Alcoholics Anonymous groups. The other half were told, in effect: 'We're glad you recognize you have a drink problem. Do try to stop drinking or at least cut down. Our social worker will call or phone once a month for the next year to see how things are going and will speak with your wife as well as you. Good luck!' They were also told, using 'sympathetic and constructive terms', that 'responsibility for attainment of the stated goals lay in their own hands rather than it being anything that could be taken over by others'. No medication or counselling was offered. If problems persisted or arose, they should contact their GP. After 12 months, there were no statistically significant differences between the groups. Nearly half had stopped drinking or were drinking much less but the 'advice' group spent less time in hospital and off work.

One explanation for such lasting changes is that the significant placebo and non-specific effects of a therapeutic intervention may persist for many years for the same reasons that, as discussed earlier, a newly-created religion or sect may remain in existence for many centuries. That is, if the intervention or creation happens at an auspicious time in the narrative of a disease, a community or an era. Apart from placebo and non-specific factors, the clinician can only guess at other reasons for these lasting cures. The patient may not be able to explain them either but sometimes, with the benefit of hindsight, it is possible to tease out a candidate or two. For example, the sudden improvements in optimism or morale that may follow exposure to a new healer, a new treatment or a new relic may enable patients to achieve some small goal that has been beyond their ability or even beyond their imagining for months or years. That in turn may enable them to adopt a different and more hopeful view of their condition and its previously assumed limitations. These things also happen spontaneously, or at any rate without any obvious explanation. Falling in love and remaining there for long enough to matter can have similar effects.

'Treatment vs Advice' also illustrates an extremely important point about both placebos and compliance, because while good compliance with treatment (i.e. diligently following 'doctor's orders') leads to better outcomes than half-hearted compliance or leaving treatment, compliance itself, *even to placebos*, is a very important predictor of good outcomes. In other words, the nature of the treatment complied with may be much less important than whether the level of compliance with treatment is high or low, probably because good compliers tend to be conscientious, diligent, health-conscious and well-organised people.[327]These personality traits are useful in most areas of life and are likely to facilitate recovery from any illness, condition or misfortune. In contrast, poor compliers are more likely to be disorganised and short on self-discipline, which is not helpful if you are trying to lose old habits and learn new ones. That is true whether the new habit is getting used to speaking a second language or getting used to not drinking.

In some respects, the beneficial effects of simply being in treatment may be similar to the Hawthorne Effect, first described in the 1920s. Psychologists were interested in how small changes in the working conditions at the Hawthorne factory that produced electrical goods, such as better lighting, might improve or impair output. To their surprise, they found that output improved almost regardless of the changes. They concluded that when people are aware of being the subject of an experiment or of simply being observed more closely than usual, their behaviour changes. In a medical context, that often means that patients respond, consciously or otherwise, in ways that they believe will please their doctors. That is a non-specific effect but like other non-specific effects, it can bias the results of studies and needs to be allowed for in their analysis. Especially in non-medical settings, the Hawthorne Effect can be eliminated by ensuring that subjects are unaware that they are taking part in an experiment. Conversely, when the object of a study is not how patients respond to treatment but, for example, how social workers, civil servants or physiotherapists do their job, it is hardly surprising that they tend to be on their best behaviour. That explains why programmes that are found to be effective in controlled trials may be ineffective, or less effective, in real life.

Placebo and non-specific effects can evidently be powerful as well as persistent. They sometimes help a larger proportion of patients in controlled trials than the specific pharmacological actions of genuinely effective drugs, especially in the case of antidepressants. It is therefore important to know whether conventional physicians could consistently exploit these effects to improve treatment outcomes. The challenge is to do this in ways that maintain or improve trust and do not damage the doctor-patient relationship. Deliberately using placebo drugs and procedures often means some deception of our patients, if only temporarily, though open-label placebos (see below) largely avoid that. In placebo-controlled randomized controlled trials, patients are told that they *might* (or might not) receive a placebo but are not usually told when the trial is over whether they were in the placebo or active group. Certainly, using open-label placebos need not and must not mean deceiving ourselves as clinicians. That is what would distinguish the ethical use of placebos by medically qualified 'non-alternative' healers from the way they are used by most CAM practitioners, as well as by sharks and charlatans. Ethicists have different views about using placebos in this way. A paper published before specific placebo research really got going argued that placebo effects didn't even exist[328] but ten years later, Prof. Jeremy Howick, a leading British placebo researcher concluded in a Cochrane-style review of published research that placebo effects are indeed real and powerful and the overwhelming majority of placebo research backs him up.[329] The debate sometimes involves complex statistical arguments that I must leave to the statisticians but the nay-sayers have very little support. There is also a growing and respectable body of argument that it can be both ethical and useful to use open-label placebos,[330] though many doctors still use impure or, less commonly, pure placebos as my generation did, despite ethical concerns. Since in practice, it is evidently impossible to ban the prescribing of placebos and quasi-placebos by physicians, surely we should at least study how best to maximise their benefits and minimize their philosophical and ethical harms which, in the management of individual patients, may turn out to be largely theoretical. One way in which conventional doctors (mainly GPs) get away with using pure placebos is to combine evidence-based orthodox medicines with relatively harmless CAM ones like homoeopathic medicines or acupuncture, knowing or presuming that they are placebos with no specific healing effects. As we'll see, that is what King Charles' rather interesting Buckingham Palace GP recently admitted.

Today's placebo researchers are increasingly studying the long-neglected evidence that people can respond positively to placebo medicines and procedures *even when they are told that they contain no active constituents,* i.e. open-label placebos.[331] A trial of open-label vs 'deceptive' placebos for pain, appropriately titled 'If only they knew!',[332] found that both were equally effective. Other studies have found deceptive, 'blinded' placebos more effective for pain[333] but 'sales techniques' can greatly influence the size of both placebo and non-specific effects and thus of subjective outcomes. Furthermore, it is the generally non-lethal chronic, distressing and often painful conditions with subjective complaints but not much in the way of abnormal tests or other objective findings that that take up so much time and money in both general and hospital out-patient practice. A recent British survey[334] noted that:

> "despite its counter-intuitive and paradoxical character, there is an increasingly robust evidence base for the use of open label placebo to treat a range of chronic conditions, including chronic low back pain, cancer-related fatigue and irritable bowel syndrome. Meta-analyses have demonstrated medium to large effects in clinical samples".

There are no blood tests or MRI scans that can explain why one patient with severe arthritis or heart disease is cheerful and active within the objective limitations of the disease, while another with the same condition is miserable and largely immobile. A 2018 BBC TV series followed a group of patients with chronic back pain, some of them in wheelchairs, who were told they might receive placebo capsules or a powerful new pain-killer. The capsules were an impressive blue and white rather than plain but all of them contained only rice powder. It therefore involved some deception but as with Prof. Ernst's actors or non-existent faith-healers, many patients improved, discontinued morphine and other potent opiate analgesics or abandoned their wheelchairs.[335] Reality can be a confusing thing. Perhaps that is one reason why mankind finds it difficult to bear very much of it.

My own experience, like that of Prof Kaptchuk and his team, indicates that debriefing individual patients who have improved with placebo treatments can be therapeutically and educationally useful. It doesn't take much time but provided that qualified doctors are in charge of diagnosis, much of the labour could be done by less expensively trained clinicians working as part of a stable and consistent team. Open-label placebos certainly cause less ethical angst among doctors than the covert kind. However, I concede immediately that these suggestions might turn out not to be useful on a larger scale in the daily practice of medicine. Even if they were shown to be useful, it might not be organizationally possible. Formidable forces might be marshalled against the idea and spearheading the attack would probably be the pharmaceutical industry, for whom placebo effects, like the null hypothesis, are an unwelcome spectre at their corporate feasts. They are already worried enough, after losing millions on developing drugs, especially drugs for unhappiness and anxiety, that failed to out-perform placebos, to have allegedly "formed a secret committee to compare all their own trial results to determine what is happening and why the effect of 'dummy' drugs is increasing".[336] We know how ruthless and dishonest some companies can be, though there are several public-spirited and generous exceptions. It seems unlikely that they would fund much placebo research aimed at reducing the demand for treatment with their products.

I suggest three broad avenues of study. First, clinical research might usefully start with disorders like irritable bowel syndrome (IBS) and other chronic pain syndromes that cause significant distress to patients, have no obvious or consistent medical cause and often do not respond well to conventional treatments. There are many patients of this kind in nearly all fields of medicine. Because this group of disorders is, almost by definition, never fatal, joining with patients in collaborative placebo research would be very unlikely to cause life-threatening exacerbations. Kaptchuk-style debriefings might provide beneficial insights and techniques for both individual patients and larger groups. Since pain is a prominent symptom in many medical consultations, research should look at the potential of hypnosis (including self-hypnosis) for making it disappear or at least become more manageable. After all, if a new analgesic drug enabled patients to tolerate with equanimity levels of pain equivalent to sitting in an ice-bath for several minutes and with no serious side effects or risk of addiction, as hypnosis clearly can, it would make its inventor and manufacturer very rich. Hypnosis seems to be closely linked to the psychological processes that mediate placebo effects and therefore hypnosis research may well make important contributions to our understanding of placebos and our ability to exploit them. It may also attract clinicians and researchers who are uncomfortable with the deceptive aspects of placebo treatment because hypnosis generally involves suggestion but not deception.

Secondly, research might explore the possible clinical applications of Terror Management Theory; the idea that, as the playwright Samuel Beckett put it, "Everything that man does in his symbolic world is an attempt to deny and overcome his grotesque fate" and what TS Eliot presumably meant by that "one end, which is always present". Or in Dr Johnson's version (and he was clearly terrified by the prospect) "All of life is but keeping away the thoughts of death". If so many people are affected in significant and measurable ways by subliminal reminders of death, as Terror Management Theory research consistently shows, perhaps we can devise ways of helping both individual patients and society in general to cope rather better with the inescapable facts of human vulnerability and mortality. That in turn might help patients to cope better with conditions like IBS, as well as more disabling illnesses caused by diseased and malfunctioning organs and it might shed additional light on placebo processes.

Thirdly, although this is only indirectly related to placebo research, it might be useful to study more general ways of helping today's future adults to become more psychologically robust. I have mentioned the steady increase in consultations and sickness benefits for psychological problems that has occurred despite an equally steady expansion of counselling and antidepressant prescribing Whatever the causes, the trend should worry us for philosophical, social and political reasons as well as for health-economic ones.

Our personalities, and thus the ways in which we respond to illness and discomfort among other challenges, do not usually change much after we pass our first quarter-century. If these trends in depression and anxiety continue, clinicians may in a couple of decades find their workloads even further increased as today's many twenty-somethings whose hopes and ambitions have not come anywhere near to being realized try to come to terms with the near-certainty that they never will be. If society encourages the young to believe that they can be anything they want to be, it arguably has a duty to pick up the pieces when many of them find that the reality is very different. Perhaps, as the philosopher Alan de Botton suggests, our museums might usefully be rearranged, with galleries that address "the concerns of our souls ... spaces that would each try to remind us in a sensory way – with the help of unapologetic labels and catalogues – of important ideas related to a number of problematic areas of our lives".[337]

Placebo research will certainly be interesting and varied as well as clinically important, whatever it reveals. Apart from medicine and psychology, researchers will need to be familiar with aspects of philosophy, anthropology, trans-cultural studies, drama, comparative theology, archaeology and salesmanship. Neuroscientists are already trying to understand how placebo effects work at a neuroanatomical and neurophysiological level and some of them will hope to find new drugs or procedures that would mimic or augment them. I wish them luck but I think that they are unlikely to discover much information that will be useful to clinicians in their daily encounters with patients. Whatever those placebo mechanisms are, they clearly have very large individual and even idiosyncratic components that reflect the enormous range of human experiences and their interpretation, context, symbolism and meaning. That contrasts sharply with the relatively crude and undiscriminating effects of the limited range of drugs we prescribe for the ever-expanding list of psychiatric diagnoses. The fictional Macbeth put this despairing question to his wife's GP:

> 'Canst thou not minister to a mind diseased,
> Pluck from the memory a rooted sorrow,
> Raze out the written troubles of the brain
> And with some sweet oblivious antidote
> Cleanse the stuffed bosom of that perilous stuff
> Which weighs upon the heart?'

A thousand years later, the answer remains, on the whole, 'I'm afraid not', unless we are dealing with a mind truly diseased by something like schizophrenia, temporal lobe epilepsy or manic-depressive illness. These days, we can easily give the world's Lady Macbeths a decent night's sleep but they must wake up eventually and in the end, they must come to terms with unpleasant realities. We probably take too many orthodox medicines and for different reasons, both the pharmaceutical industry and doctors in general underestimate the incidence of side effects but this is particularly true of the drugs used in psychiatry that are intended to alter the way that patients feel and think. We certainly take far too many antidepressant and anti-anxiety drugs. For most recipients, NICE (the National Institute for Health and Care Excellence) agrees that antidepressants confer very minimal benefits compared with placebos while costing the NHS a lot of money and causing significant amounts of harm from side effects, interactions with other medication and suicidal overdoses.

To encourage patients to be much more aware of the importance of psychological factors and placebo effects in many illnesses and in virtually all CAM treatments, the public as well as clinicians would need to enter into an informed debate. That would surely upset most of the CAM industry because a debate based on high-quality evidence, rather than claims from CAM practitioners with large and obvious financial axes to grind or *ex cathedra* assertions from Buckingham Palace, would mean official endorsement of the conclusion that almost all their treatments are placebos whose real or apparent effects have nothing to do with the theories that underlie them. An endorsement of that kind would not inevitably mean that patients would stop using CAM. I said in the Introduction that neither CAM nor religion are about to disappear but as I will shortly argue might occur with religion, the users of CAM might come to see it in a different light and use it in a different way. If that, in turn, made CAM practitioners stop making absurd claims for the specific effectiveness of their treatments and stop talking about meridians, potencies, *doshas,* magnets, royal jelly and *zang-fu,* it would be a helpful start to the debate. By a happy coincidence, while I was writing this chapter, Dr Michael Dixon, the head of the medical household at Buckingham Palace, seemed to be doing exactly that in an interview for *The Times*.[338]

Now in his 70s, he has worked in a busy NHS practice in semi-rural Devon and in many ways, he sounds like the sort of GP that most patients would like to have. For a start, he and his partners offer the continuity of care which, as he recognizes but today's NHS apparently doesn't, can reduce mortality and morbidity by over 10%,[339] a larger reduction than some widely-used effective drugs achieve. "Too often you ask patients who their GP is and they don't know. We've lost that connection, which is fundamental. Yesterday, having been in the same practice for 40 years, I saw the grandchildren of patients I've known all that time, and the children that I delivered. It made it easier for me, because I knew the family. We know that if GPs have an ongoing relationship with the patient, you refer less, you prescribe less, and they go to hospital less." His practice also works with local organisations to encourage non-pharmacological 'social prescribing' like volunteering or referring patients for art classes, gardening and singing groups, which must be easier in a small community with strong social links. He believes it is "madness" that 20% of adults in the UK are on antidepressants. Me too. "If you only have five or ten minutes per appointment, it's far easier for me to give you Prozac than to start talking about life stresses, work and all the rest of it". Every British GP shares his despair at the massive increase in paperwork, box-ticking and "mandatory NHS training on topics including fire safety, equality and diversity and preventing terrorist radicalization ... We're infantilised as professionals." So far, so uncontroversial.

What is really striking about the interview, though, is that Dixon is chair of the College of Medicine, the misleadingly orthodox-sounding title of what was originally a CAM pressure-group. It insisted on the specific effectiveness of CAM treatments and had links with the then Prince Charles, who had regularly called for more research into CAM since the 1980s. The Prince should, therefore, have been delighted when Prof. Edzard Ernst was appointed to head the world's first university department intended to do just that, because Prof. Ernst's entire remit was to find out whether CAM treatments had any specific therapeutic effects beyond placebo and non-specific ones. Having worked after qualifying at one of Germany's surprisingly numerous homoeopathic hospitals, he had not been hostile to homoeopathy but then worked in another field before a mid-life career-change. When his careful researches revealed that homoeopathy and nearly all other CAM interventions had no convincing advantage over comparable placebos, the Prince became very angry and Prof. Ernst was edged out of his chair. His numerous differences with the CAM-loving prince are amusingly detailed in his autobiography[340] and his latest book.[341] A decade before Prof. Ernst took up his post at Exeter University, I wrote an article that criticised Prince Charles for giving a kind of royal 'By Appointment' cachet to CAM. It ended:

> "It is ironic that [royals] seem to be so unaware of the power of the placebo effect since they are, in a sense, its walking incarnation. What else is the placebo effect except respect, suggestibility, image, tradition, expectation and good publicity? What else is the monarchy? That is why both of them can be so useful.... Good royals, like good doctors, can give a powerfully comforting feeling that all is well when to the objective observer, the reality is rather depressing. Some people believe in Santa Claus. Not all of them are children."[342]

Although Dr Dixon denies having ever studied homoeopathy, or used it, he has said that "if patients feel they've benefited from homeopathy, what's the problem?" Even if the theory behind the treatment is absurd, if it helps his patients that is all that matters. "I didn't care a damn if it's placebo; they got better." Another way of putting this unashamed confession would be: "I recommend and prescribe treatments that I know or believe are placebos and have no specific effect *but I don't tell the patients that.*" Which is exactly what all doctors, including me, quite often did until the 1970s for both therapeutic and diagnostic reasons. Evidently many doctors still do in a more hesitant but still deceptive and sometimes needlessly expensive way. If deceptive placebo prescribing is now completely unethical, that could and possibly should mean stern letters from the General Medical Council to those doctors, particularly to Dr Dixon. Conversely, if it isn't unethical, the GMC should say so, or at least indicate the clinical scenarios in which it might be permissible.

In this respect, Dixon's apostasy, if that term describes it correctly, is not an isolated case. A small but increasing number of CAM practitioners are responding to criticism by saying: "Yes, of course homoeopathy, acupuncture, cupping and what have you are all placebos but it's obvious that placebos can be very powerful, so why should we stop? Especially since, unlike some of your orthodox drugs and procedures, most of them do little or no serious harm; and many patients like them".[343] One obvious and serious objection to this argument is that most CAM practitioners have no training in medicine. More than qualified doctors, they can and do ignore or misdiagnose serious and treatable illness. They may also advise patients to discontinue even life-saving drugs. In December 2024, a CAM practitioner of 'slapping therapy' was given a ten-year prison sentence after advising an insulin-dependent diabetic to stop her insulin, causing her rapid decline and death. That is not true of experienced and properly trained doctors like Dr Dixon who also use CAM, however deviously. They are in a similar category to the more medically-respected doctors who use hypnosis, which Dr Dixon also does. In any case, CAM is often used in addition to orthodox medicine when a diagnosis has already been made. That is presumably why it is called 'complementary'. Sometimes it may simply represent a hedging of bets, like the Jamaicans who received state-of-the-art treatment at the university hospital and also sacrificed chickens with an obeah-man, but it may also reflect the limitations of even the best orthodox treatment, especially in the many conditions where social and psychological factors powerfully influence the level of distress and discomfort. I am emphatically not trying to encourage more use of CAM but I do think that orthodox physicians could benefit from a greater understanding of the reasons why so many of their patients use CAM and of the psychological mechanisms that enable patients to say that they feel better after it (and therefore, incidentally, perhaps spend less time in GP waiting rooms and on hospital waiting lists). They might also benefit from understanding why patients often strongly prefer one type of CAM over alternative 'Alternative' procedures. Meanwhile, let us hope for his sake that Dr Dixon's high-profile dismissal of CAM's potencies, succussions, psora, auras, needles, meridians and specific effectiveness survives royal displeasure. If he always tells his patients that the CAM treatments he advises are placebos and have no specific effects but may relieve symptoms like other open-label placebos, we can hardly complain. However, it is ironic, and vaguely annoying, that the only practitioners in the healing business who can currently use placebos deceptively without any professional comeback are the healers with no medical training who mostly insist that the placebos they use and recommend are amazingly effective remedies; that, as with the late Steve Jobs, their CAM treatments for cancer are as good as current anti-cancer drugs; or that Africa's "ancient traditional knowledge", praised by Dr Tshabalala-Msimang, is as effective as HAART for her country's numerous HIV-infected citizens. All this and more despite an Everest of evidence that they are no such thing.

If open-label placebos are to be studied and used more often, the likely reluctance of many doctors to behave in ways that involve playing a role or simulating sincerity could be an obstacle. Using and manipulating placebo effects, even when the aim is to demonstrate the importance of psychological processes to the patient, as with the Kaptchuk debriefing study and my sham-ECT patient, may involve being economical with the truth and even if doctors and clinical psychologists were prepared to do that, they might not be very good at it. Maximising success in augmenting and 'selling' placebo effects requires thespian skills – the same simulated sincerity and enthusiasm that leading thespians are generously paid to deploy when they do voice-overs for advertisements. So I have a suggestion: why not use *real* thespians in open-label placebo research? Prof. Ernst used actors in his spiritual healing study with impressive results. Prof Kaptchuk greatly boosted the beneficial effects of placebo acupuncture in Irritable Bowel Syndrome by that 'augmented' consultation that he described unashamedly as "at least 20 minutes of very schmaltzy care ('I'm so glad to meet you...I know how difficult this is for you...This treatment has excellent results')" during which "Practitioners were also required to touch the hands or shoulders of [patients in the 'augmented'] group and spend at least 20 seconds lost in thoughtful silence".[344] This scripted and impersonal intervention clearly felt insincere to the clinicians involved but it significantly improved the outcome; and sincerity is what actors train for years to simulate and perfect. (As Marlon Brando is said to have admitted: "Lying for a living. That's what acting is".)[345] They can 'do' sincerity better than most doctors and counsellors and probably for less money since, unlike doctors, many of them are under-employed or unemployed. Plus, you can't overdose on thespians.

However, Artificial Intelligence may already have made this only slightly tongue-in-cheek suggestion irrelevant because robot therapists, programmed to emit convincing, Kaptchuk-style insincerities,[346] are already able to do the job. Computerised 'interpretations' may satisfy patients as much as those made by human therapists and computerised cognitive-behavioural therapy for depression seems to be of comparable effectiveness to the face-to-face variety.[347] "AI is capable of acting as a confidant, an adviser, a therapist, a non-judgmental friend ... Loneliness is a great human evil. Lonely people die younger, and severe loneliness can lead to self-harm or suicide. Now we have machines which can probably solve much of this overnight."[348] Similar developments have occurred in religion. What may be the first robot priest has already been wheeled-out in Wittenberg, the town where Luther initiated the Reformation in 1517 by supposedly nailing his 39 theses to the door of the *Schlosskirche*. "The Protestant Church in Germany has unveiled a robotic priest called BlessU-2 to mark 500 years since the Reformation. The machine delivers various blessings in eight languages."[349] The report notes that Luther, too, made extensive use of the new technology of his day: printing. If open label placebo research involves CAM therapies, actors could be trained to do most of those as well, with little difficulty. As many RCTs have shown, doing acupuncture the 'right' way according to the sacred texts of CAM is either unimportant or very much less important than impressive sales-talk and that is probably true for almost the whole of CAM. I would expect suitably trained actors to make rather good CAM therapists and they would not have to bear the weight of therapeutic delusions. Many actors already act as pseudo-patients, on whom medical students can learn their craft without clumsily upsetting real patients and making them even more anxious. When the 26th of the Church of England's 39 Articles notes that "The sacraments are effectual because of Christ's institution and promise, even though they may be administered by evil men", it is effectively saying that even if parishioners have grave doubts or only very basic faith, the setting, the scenery and the sales-talk are more important than the technical details – the 'content', if you like – of that faith.

To the objection that insincerity is fundamentally wrong and unethical, there are several responses. One is that certain types of insincerity, including some important examples of what we call 'social skills', are essential for the continuation and smooth running of most human relationships, including doctor-patient ones. I enjoyed being a doctor and can honestly say that I never had a day when I wished I had chosen some other profession but all doctors have a few patients who test their tolerance and simulated sincerity to the limits. Another is to remember Jean Meslier, the village priest who spent his entire professional life insincerely reciting the prayers and benedictions that he privately deplored but that he knew gave comfort and reassurance to his parishioners. There is no evidence that either he or they suffered any serious psychological or spiritual damage during those decades of benevolent deception. In any case, debriefing people who have responded to placebos clearly provides opportunities to persuade them that they are much more resilient than they realised. It might even enable them to discontinue medicines that they do not need and that are sometimes toxic. It bears repeating that antidepressants are a classic and collectively very costly example.

2: Religion.

While I hope this book has been interesting and thought-provoking, I don't expect it to cause much head-nodding among religious people who are convinced of the truth of their religious beliefs and not interested in questioning them. Fortunately, there is a spectrum of religious belief ranging from certainty to serious doubt and I hope it will interest those on the middle and questioning parts of that spectrum. (Agnostics also inhabit a spectrum but in practice, many of them seem to live their daily lives much like definite atheists.) In particular, I hope that if they accept the idea that religion has much in common with placebo and non-specific effects, it will persuade them that religions themselves have so much in common that enmity between them, let alone violence, should be unthinkable.

To these believers, I would say that it does not necessarily mean you should stop practising your own religion. Continuing to practise it for other reasons, as many practising Anglicans and Catholics in Britain do, need not involve either abandoning every ancient tradition, or serious intellectual dishonesty. You should just go very easy on the truth-claims. To put it another way, just as people can respond well to open-label placebos even when they know that that they are placebos, what it seems appropriate to call 'open-label religion' – the ritual, symbolic and social features without the doctrines and truth-claims – may substitute very satisfactorily for the full-fat, deity-enriched version. If you've already gone easy on the truth claims and particularly if you worry about the afterlife and your place in it, consider letting go of them altogether. Like 'true' needles in acupuncture or 'true' dilutions and succussions of homoeopathic medicines, they are nothing like as important as religious leaders (or your mother) say they are. Active membership of a church can confer benefits but so can active involvement in almost any group, including the non-religious Sunday gatherings that have become popular in some circles, the many non-religious helping and volunteering organisations and, of course, hobby-groups. Just as elaborate treatment rituals usually have bigger placebo effects than simpler ones, elaborate religious rituals may be more satisfying than the plainer kind but the choice of ritual is a matter of taste that really has no specific consequences, just as placebos have no specific effects; and to say that is not to devalue either ritual or placebos. We have seen that it does not matter to his or her parishioners if the priest in charge secretly rejects the underlying doctrines and that even open rejection of them may not alienate a congregation. Of course, religion can have an important role as a badge of cultural identity and as a comforting but – according to Albert Einstein, Isaiah Berlin and many other thoughtful and well-read people – evidence-free way of dealing with fundamental existential questions like the meaning and purpose of life and what happens after we die. However, in a society of many cultures, it seems undesirable to prioritise the one characteristic of religion – its insistence on truth-claims - that has led to so many particularly pointless feuds, wars and massacres and that has seen a worrying recent revival of them in the streets, transport systems and concert halls of Britain and several other Western countries, as well as much bloodier ones between competing Muslim sects.

In any case, where Britain's national, Established church is concerned, many senior Anglicans have said things in print that are not very different from what I have just written. Sixty years ago, *Honest to God*, a best-selling book by the Bishop of Woolwich, John Robinson, argued very publicly that the supernatural concept of God was outdated, simplistic and, in short, wrong. Several commentators soon pointed out that he wasn't saying anything very new. What annoyed many churchmen and parishioners at the time was that he had been tactless enough to make public the divergence between the everyday Christianity of hymns, ritual, prayers, sermons, good works and flower-arranging and the much more rarefied, less ritualistic and less earthy Christianity that was regularly discussed at seminars, lectures, retreats and dinners in deaneries and theological colleges throughout the land but decently out of hearing of the faithful. As theologian and former priest Don Cupitt wrote in a volume commemorating the 40th anniversary of Honest to God:

> "There is the common ecclesiastical faith to which [priests] are institutionally committed, and which they must unhesitatingly defend in public; and there is the personal faith to which they have been led by their own study and thinking. Every church leader who is theologically educated is aware of the gap between the two, and of the devices that must be used to conceal it".[350]

Sixty years on, it seems that many church-goers have bridged that gap by maintaining the comforting and familiar rituals, while accommodating and adapting to post-Robinsonian doubts and doctrinal reconfigurations. In his televised 'Miracle' stage performance, the openly atheist Derren Brown demonstrates that the classic techniques and rituals of Evangelical faith-healing could be used successfully even after a blasphemous and satirical audience warm-up that would have got the show instantly banned by the Lord Chamberlain, before his role as theatrical censor was abolished in 1968.

There are people in all countries for whom religion is a crucial and fundamental part of their life and their identity. In some countries, that describes all or most citizens but for many European countries from the mid-20th century until a few decades ago, it generally described a small and declining minority. Today, the dichotomy between the religiously tolerant and unbelieving or indifferent majority and the small but probably growing minority of fervent, intolerant and exclusivist sectarians is an increasing cause of concern and friction, because religious doctrines affect not only the way people live their own lives but also the way they behave towards neighbours who don't share their faith. As a secularist, I have no wish to tell these devoutly religious people how to practise their religion but as a British (and European) secularist, one of my subsidiary aims is to remind everyone who lives here, regardless of their faith or ethnicity, of some important historical trends and events that we seem in danger of forgetting. In Britain, as in all European countries and many non-European ones, the right to practise your religion freely goes with a corresponding right to change or criticise your religion, the right not to have a religion and the right to criticise the fundamental beliefs of other faiths or of theism in general, just as religious people have an equal right to criticise the arguments of unbelievers. Most religions also embody ideas about how society should be ordered, as do all political parties. The right to freely and openly criticise religious beliefs, institutions and proposals is therefore part of the right to criticise political ones. Those rights are fundamental for democracy and have been hard won over several centuries. Many people suffered and died for them and although they are incorporated into the Universal Declaration of Human Rights, they are once again in danger, notably from countries like Saudi Arabia, and their growing diasporas, that never agreed to sign that part of the Declaration when it was unveiled after the ideological slaughters of WW2. In the long run, it might help social cohesion in Europe if the less fanatical believers could persuade the leaders of their own faiths to declare that they unequivocally accept and support these rights. It is unlikely that this book will be published or openly sold in Islamic countries, or in a Russia where the Russian Orthodox Church is once again a power in the land. In an open letter published two days before he died in the *Charlie Hebdo* massacre of 2015, its editor and cartoonist had written: "In France, a religion is nothing more than a collection of texts, traditions, and customs that it is perfectly legitimate to criticize". I would have added 'beliefs' to that collection.

When State and Church were much more closely linked than they are today in the West, accepting the concept of freedom of religious belief did not immediately mean that nobody suffered any sanctions for refusing to follow the dominant creed but it did gradually come to mean that nobody lost their life or their liberty for being a dissenter. Unbelievers were the last of the major dissenters to be admitted to Parliament, in 1886, long after Catholics (1829) and Jews (1848) but Westminster now accommodates several dozen at least, without obvious problems. In the USA, an avowed unbeliever might find it difficult to get elected to Congress in many areas but unbelief is not illegal and the 'nones' are now growing faster than those who identify as having a religion. From its foundation, the USA has had strong and generally effective legislation that created what Thomas Jefferson,[351] one of the Founding Fathers of the USA and its third president, famously called 'a wall of separation' between Church and State. In a pre-Darwinian world, it is not surprising that Jefferson subscribed to the almost universal belief in an afterlife but where this world was concerned, he was a deist close to the Spinoza-Voltaire-Einstein variety and he was relaxed about unbelief, noting that "it does me no injury for my neighbour to say there are twenty gods, or no god. It neither picks my pocket nor breaks my leg". He admired some of the philosophical and political ideas attributed to Jesus but rejected all the supernatural and miraculous aspects of Christianity, writing to his fellow-President John Adams that "the day will come, when the mystical generation of Jesus, by the Supreme Being as His Father, in the womb of a virgin, will be classed with the fable of the generation of Minerva, in the brain of Jupiter." He may never have read Meslier's *Testament* but in words that Meslier himself could have written, Jefferson criticised the clergy for using religion as a "mere contrivance to filch wealth and power to themselves".

Prominent clerics regularly complain that secularism is synonymous with militant, proselytizing atheism. In reality, all it means is the sort of Jeffersonian Church-State separation that the drafters of the First Amendment to the Constitution thought to be so important for the future stability of the new republic:

"Congress shall make no law respecting an establishment of religion, or prohibiting the free exercise thereof; or abridging the freedom of speech, or of the press; or the right of the people peaceably to assemble, and to petition the Government for a redress of grievances."

Jefferson's immediate predecessor, John Adams, proclaimed that "... the government of the United States is not, in any sense, founded on the Christian religion; ... [It]is not a Christian nation any more than it is a Jewish or a Mohammedan nation".[352] A few years later, Jefferson wrote that:

"We have solved, by fair experiment, the great and interesting question whether freedom of religion is compatible with order in government and obedience to the laws. And we have experienced the quiet as well as the comfort which results from leaving every one to profess freely and openly those principles of religion which are the inductions of his own reason and the serious convictions of his own inquiries."

He urged his fellow-Americans to "Fix Reason firmly in her seat, and call to her tribunal every fact, every opinion. Question with boldness even the existence of a God". Neither the null hypothesis nor the placebo effect had been specifically formulated in Jefferson's time but I think that he would have enthusiastically endorsed both ideas, as well as the idea of God and religion as cosmic placebos.

Acknowledgements

Michael Aubrey wrote perceptive marginal comments typical of a former Head of English. Dr Justin Basquille kept me in touch with current psychiatric practices and fashions. Dr Julian Bird, psychiatrist and professional actor, shared his international expertise on psychosomatic problems and, together with Daniel Simpson, tried to convince me that thespians are not experts in insincerity. Dr Leslie Brann, Derren Brown, Prof Michael Heap and Robert Welfare enlarged my understanding of hypnosis. Prof David Denney and Prof David Smith supplied helpful sociological insights. Prof Jacalyn Duffin discussed her research on saints and miracles in the Vatican archives. Dr Mark Hockey and Dr Dow Smith recalled some challenging psychosomatic patients. Prof Edzard Ernst and Nick Ross persuaded me not to encourage research into the deceptive use of placebos. John Illman and Karl Sabbagh provided editorial advice. Dr George O'Neil, a former missionary obstetrician in Africa who now runs an exemplary high-tech, low-cost addiction clinic in Perth, enabled me to observe the soothing effects of his prayers on a patient undergoing heroin withdrawal. Over the years, several other religious friends, including Dr Steve Kelly, Tom Longford, Dean Andrew Nunn, the late Philippe Pillorget, Dr Mark Pickering of the Christian Medical Fellowship and the late Dean Colin Slee have informed my views on religion and its rituals. Some commented on early drafts or tried to persuade me of the authenticity of Biblical accounts and Mary Snowden offered the perspective of someone who nearly became a nun. Keith Porteous-Wood of the National Secular Society and Prof Clive Coen of the Rationalist Association (now merged once more with HumanistsUK) encouraged me from the other side of the religious fence. James Loader answered literary questions and Sebastian Payne contributed his constitutional lawyer's eye for detail. Dr. Erin Kelty tracked down several obscure sources. Jeffrey Masson added to his accounts of dirty work in the Freud archives. Dr Andrew Willis shared my recollections of placebo use at a time when morale in the NHS was high despite our therapeutic limitations. Dr Emmanuel Streel, my co-author in several papers about addiction, has never let our friendship impair his academic rigour. Daniel Dennett and I exchanged a single email. My contact with Richard Dawkins extended no further than once shaking hands with him and I never met or communicated with Sam Harris but the writings of all three affect any current discussion about the origins, evolution, uses and abuses of religion. The quotation from T S

Eliot's *Burnt Norton* is reproduced by permission of Faber and Co. Finally, as well as lamenting the decline of NHS general practice, my imperturbable partner provided untiring support, encouragement and humour, putting up with nocturnal typing and occasional voice memos or requests to remind me when I feared I might forget a usable inspiration by the morning.

Notes and References

[1] You can read about it on my website, planetservetus.org. Miguel Servetus, a Spanish physician and philosopher, was burned alive in 1553, together with his books, by the Protestant John Calvin because of a disagreement about the nature of the Holy Trinity.

[2] From his obituary in the N Y Times April 19th, 1955.

[3] Pirajno, Duke of. A cure for serpents: an Italian doctor in North Africa. London. Eland. 1985, 75-8.

[4] In January 2017, Kellyanne Conway, a spokesperson for the newly-elected President Trump, coined the interesting term 'alternative facts'. Previously, they had been called 'falsehoods' or 'untruths' when sincerely, if mistakenly, believed by the speaker; and 'lies' when known or strongly suspected by the speaker to be untrue.

[5] Kaptchuk T, Kerr C, Zanger A. Placebo Controls, Exorcisms and the Devil, Lancet. 2009 Oct 10; 374(9697): 1234.

[6] Until the mid 1960s, the bottles in which medicines were dispensed were usually labelled simply as 'The Tablets', The Capsules' or 'The Mixture'. This made prescribing placebos easy. By adding the initials 'NP' (nomen propria – 'own name'), prescribers could instruct the pharmacist to add the name of the drug but it was optional. Until the early 1970s, by adding 'NNP' (non nomen propria) the pharmacist could be discreetly instructed to withhold this information but eventually full labelling, and then information packs with lists of possible side effects, became mandatory. Unsurprisingly, complaints of side-effects increased considerably.

[7] Diary, 31st Dec 1664.

[8] Diary 24th Jan 1664/5

[9] Ernst E, Resch KL. Concept of true and perceived placebo effects. BMJ 1995, 311, 551-3

[10] de Botton A. religion for atheists, London, Penguin, 2012, passim

[11] Gray, J. The Immortalization Commission. London, Allen Lane 2011

[12] Except for a jokey one in the BMJ's humorous Christmas edition. The 'jump' was about half a metre from the wing of a small, stationary plane. Yeh R W, Valsdottir L R, Yeh M W. et al. Parachute use to prevent death and major trauma when jumping from aircraft: randomized controlled trial BMJ 2018; 363 :k5094 doi:10.1136/bmj.k5094

[13] https://www.theguardian.com/world/2025/jan/29/india-crowd-crush-kumbh-mela-religious-festival-death-toll-injuries-prayagraj?utm_term=6799b9561c9ae767f7a54d7eda698f98&utm_campaign=GuardianTodayUK&utm_source=esp&utm_medium=Email&CMP=GTUK_email

[14] Yadav J, Bhardwaj A, Jangid P, Singh P, Gupta R. Meditation-A Slippery Slope for Psychosis: A Case Series With Review of Evidence. J Nerv Ment Dis. 2023 Aug 1;211(8):634-638. doi: 10.1097/NMD.0000000000001656. PMID: 37505896.

[15] Cobb LA, Thomas GI, Dillard DH, Merendino KA, Bruce RA. An evaluation of internal-mammary-artery ligation by a double-blind technic. N Engl J Med 1959;260:1115-8.

[16] Leon M, Kornowski R, Downey W et al. A blinded, randomized, placebo-controlled trial of percutaneous laser myocardial revascularization to improve angina symptoms in patients with severe coronary disease. J Am Coll Cardiol. 2005 Nov 15;46(10):1812-9.

[17] Al-Lamee R, Thompson D, Dehbi HM et al Percutaneous coronary intervention in stable angina (ORBITA): a double-blind, randomised controlled trial. Lancet DOI: http://dx.doi.org/10.1016/S0140-6736(17)32714-9 |Published: 02 November 2017

[18] Buchbinder R1, Osborne RH, Ebeling PR, Wark JD, Mitchell P, Wriedt C, Graves S, Staples MP, Murphy B. A randomized trial of vertebroplasty for painful osteoporotic vertebral fractures. N Engl J Med. 2009 Aug 6;361(6):557-68. doi: 10.1056/NEJMoa0900429.

[19] Moseley JB, O'Malley K, Petersen NJ, Menke TJ, Brody BA, Kuykendall DH, et al. A controlled trial of arthroscopic surgery for osteoarthritis of the knee. N Engl J Med2002;347:81-8.

[20] Wartolowska K et al. Use of placebo controls in the evaluation of surgery: systematic review BMJ 2014;348:g3253

[21] Abbot NC, Harkness EF, Stevinson C, Marshall FP, Conn DA, Ernst E. Spiritual healing as a therapy for chronic pain: a randomized, clinical trial. Pain. 2001 Mar;91(1-2):79-89.

[22] Lock S. "O that I were young again": Yeats and the Steinach operation. Br Med J (Clin Res Ed). 1983 Dec 24-31;287(6409):1964-8.

[23] Dahl R. Galloping Foxley. The Roald Dahl Omnibus. New York. Barnes and Noble. 1993. 85

[24] Scruton R Fools, frauds and firebrands: thinkers of the new left. London. Bloomsbury. 2015. p 185.

[25] de Botton A. religion for atheists, London, Penguin, 2012, 14

[26] Interior wall plaque, Hospital of St John and St Elizabeth. London NW8. Matron, wearing the uniform of her religious order, did her rounds every evening and spoke with every conscious patient.

[27] Dennett D, LaScola L. Preachers Who Are Not Believers. Evolutionary Psychology 2010. 8(1): 122-150

[28] http://clergyproject.org/clergy-project-demographics/

[29]http://www.samharris.org/blog/item/life-without-god accessed 17 Feb 2012

[30] Darwin J. After Tamerlane: the rise and fall of global empires 1400-2000. London. Penguin. 2008. 141

[31] http://www.patheos.com/blogs/rationaldoubt/2015/03/holy-week-for-non-believing-clergy/ accessed 7 Apr 2015

[32] Shrell-Fox R. When Rabbis Lose Faith: Twelve Rabbis Tell their Stories about their Loss of Belief in God, Science, Religion and Culture, 2015, 2 (3) 131-146

[33] Article 26 of the 39 Articles of Religion

[34] Galanter M. Sprituality and the healthy mind: science, therapy and the need for personal meaning. Oxford. OUP. 2005, 214-22

[35] Vega CP. Low Back Pain Prevalent in Different Parts of the World. http://www.medscape.org/viewarticle/825885

[36] Alfred Adler was among the first of the original Viennese psychoanalytical circle to split with Freud.

[37] https://www.youtube.com/watch?v=Fmp14eSdUEI

[38] Alden P, Heap M. Hypnotic pain control: some theoretical and practical issues Int J Clin Exp Hypn. 1998 Jan;46(1):62-76.

[39] Faymonville ME, Boly M, Laureys S. Functional neuroanatomy of the hypnotic state. J Physiol Paris. 2006 Jun;99(4-6):463-9.

[40] Abrahamsen R1, Baad-Hansen L, Svensson P. Hypnosis in the management of persistent idiopathic orofacial pain--clinical and psychosocial findings. Pain. 2008 May;136(1-2):44-52.

[41] Liossi C, Hatira P. Clinical hypnosis versus cognitive behavioral training for pain management with pediatric cancer patients undergoing bone marrow aspirations. Int J Clin Exp Hypn. 1999 Apr;47(2):104-16.

[42] Montgomery GH, Bovbjerg DH, Schnur JB, et al A randomized clinical trial of a brief hypnosis intervention to control side effects in breast surgery patients. J Natl Cancer Inst. 2007 Sep 5;99(17):1304-12. Epub 2007 Aug 28.

[43] Deltito JA. Hypnosis in the treatment of acute pain in the emergency department setting. Postgrad Med J. 1984,60 263-6

[44] Meurisse M1, Faymonville ME, Joris J, et al. [Endocrine surgery by hypnosis. From fiction to daily clinical application: article in French] Ann Endocrinol (Paris). 1996;57(6):494-501.

[45] Mason A.A. A case of congenital icthyosiform erythrodermia of Brocq treated by hypnosis. Brit Med J 1952, Aug 23, 422-3

[46] Dr Josph Guillotin was also a member. Both Lavoisier and Louis XVI were executed with the machine that Guillotin, who opposed capital punishment, recommended as a humane improvement on the prevailing methods. It is said that he was so distressed by his association with the device that he changed his surname after the Revolution.

[47] Justman S. Pills in a pretty box: social sources of the placebo effect. In: In: (Eds. A Raz and C Harris) Placebo Talks. Oxford. OUP. 2016. 146-7.

[48] Best M, Neuhauser D, Slavin L. Evaluating Mesmerism, Paris, 1784: the controversy over blinded placebo controlled trials has not stopped. Quality & safety in health care 2003,12 (3): 232–3.

[49] London, Haygarth, J. On the imagination as a cause and as a cure of disorders of the body, exemplified by fictitious tractors and epidemical convulsions. London, Cadell and Davies 1801.

[50] K Wiech, M Farias, G Kahane, N Shackel, W Tiede, I Tracey (2008). An fMRI study measuring analgesia enhanced by religion as a belief system . Pain 2008. 139(2):467-76

[51] Lieberman M The neural correlates of placebo effects: a disruption account. NeuroImage, 2004. 22 (1), 447-455

[52] Moerman D. Looking at placebos through a cultural lens and finding meaning. In: (Eds. A Raz and C Harris) Placebo Talks. Oxford. OUP. 2016. 108.

[53] It was equally proud, in some quarters, of being the last London medical school to admit women and dentists. Its motto translates as: 'Of all the arts, medicine is the most brilliant'.

[54] Burch D. Digging up the Dead: Uncovering the Life and Times of an Extraordinary Surgeon (2007), London. Chatto and Windus.p. 26. thechirurgeonsapprentice.com/2011/10/04/cutting-for-the-stone-the-case-of-stephen-pollard/#f1

[55] Burney F. A Mastectomy at the hands of Baron Larrey. Fanny Burney: selected letters and journals. (Ed. Joyce Hemlow) OUP 1987 127-41

[56] Barbagli, M. Farewell to the world: a history of suicide. London, Polity 2017. 199-200.

[57] Phillips DP, Liu GC, Kwok K, Jarvinen JR, Zhang W, Abramson IS. The Hound of the Baskervilles effect: natural experiment on the influence of psychological stress on timing of death. BMJ. 2001 Dec 22-29;323(7327):1443-6. In the famous Sherlock Holmes story, the victim is frightened to death by an enormous hound made even more terrifying by luminous paint around its eyes.

[58] Brewer C. ECT: white man's magic? New Psychiatry, Nov 14th 1975, 8-9.

[59] Johnstone EC, Deakin JF, Lawler P, Frith CD, Stevens M, McPherson K, Crow TJ. The Northwick Park electroconvulsive therapy trial. Lancet. 1980 Dec 20-27;2(8208-8209):1317-20.

[60] Gillving C, Ekman CJ, Hammar Å, Landén M, Lundberg J, Movahed Rad P, Nordanskog P, von Knorring L, Nordenskjöld A. Seizure Duration and Electroconvulsive Therapy in Major Depressive Disorder. JAMA Netw Open. 2024 Jul 1;7(7):e2422738. doi: 10.1001/jamanetworkopen.2024.22738. PMID: 39052292; PMCID: PMC11273235.

[61] Read J, Harrop C, Morrison L, Hancock SP, Johnstone L, Cunliffe S. A large exploratory survey of electroconvulsive therapy recipients, family members and friends: what information do they recall being given? J Med Ethics. 2025 Aug 14:jme-2024-110629. doi: 10.1136/jme-2024-110629. Epub ahead of print. PMID: 40813058.

[62] Blease CR. Electroconvulsive therapy, the placebo effect and informed consent. J Med Ethics. 2013 Mar 39(3):166-70.

[63] Ackner, B; Harris, A; Oldham, AJ. Insulin treatment of schizophrenia; a controlled study. Lancet 1957;272 (6969): 607–11.

[64] Thuillier J (Transl. Hickish G) Ten years that changed the face of mental illness. London. Martin Dunitz. 1999. 26

[65] Ibid p 42

[66] Hale White W. Materia Medica. London. Churchill. 1905. p 233

[67] Which now houses my modest archive.

[68] A Google search gives no examples of deaths from refusal.

[69] http://www.diapedia.org/type-1-diabetes-mellitus/2104085199/natural-history

[70] Schenk LA, Fadai T, Büchel C. How side effects can improve treatment efficacy: a randomized trial. Brain. 2024 Aug 1;147(8):2643-2651. doi: 10.1093/brain/awae132. PMID: 38701224.

[71] Phillips DP, Liu GC, Kwok K, Jarvinen JR, Zhang W, Abramson IS. The Hound of the Baskervilles effect: natural experiment on the influence of psychological stress on timing of death. BMJ. 2001 Dec 22-29;323(7327):1443-6. In the Sherlock Holmes novel of the same name, Sir Charles Baskerville dies of a heart attack when confronted with a mastiff made additionally terrifying by local legend and the application of luminous paint by the villain of the story who hopes to inherit the estate.

[72] Syquia F C. Exorcism. Encounters with the paranormal and occult. Quezon City. Shepherd's Voice Publications. 2006, 245

[73] Wilkinson T. The Vatican's Exorcists. Driving out the Devil in the 21st century. NY. Warner. 2007, 74.

[74] Ibid. 57

[75] From memory. It's from the 1960s and I've not been able to track down the reference

[76] Faria V, Gingnell M, Hoppe JM, Hjorth O, Alaie I, Frick A, Hultberg S, Wahlstedt K, Engman J, Månsson KNT, Carlbring P, Andersson G, Reis M, Larsson EM, Fredrikson M, Furmark T. Do You Believe It? Verbal Suggestions Influence the Clinical and Neural Effects of Escitalopram in Social Anxiety Disorder: A Randomized Trial. EBioMedicine. 2017 Oct;24:179-188. doi: 10.1016/j.ebiom.2017.09.031. Epub 2017 Sep 27. PMID: 29033138; PMCID: PMC5652281.

[77] Jensen JS, Bielefeldt AØ, Hróbjartsson A. Active placebo control groups of pharmacological interventions were rarely used but merited serious

consideration: a methodological overview. J Clin Epidemiol. 2017 Jul;87:35-46. doi: 10.1016/j.jclinepi.2017.03.001. Epub 2017 Mar 22. PMID: 28342907.

[78] Heaton-Ward WA. Inference and Suggestion in a Clinical Trial (Niamid in Mongolism) Brit J Psychiat Nov 1962, 108 (457) 865-870;

[79] Cuijpers P, Cristea IA. What if placebo effect explained all the activity of depression treatments? World Psychiat 2015; 14, 310-11.

[80] Opoliner A, Azrael D, Barber C, et al.: Explaining geographic patterns of suicide in the US: the role of firearms and antidepressants. Inj Epidemiol 2014 Dec 1 (1):6.

[81] Le Noury J et al. Restoring Study 329: efficacy and harms of paroxetine and imipramine in treatment of major depression in adolescence. BMJ 2015;351:h4320 www.bmj.com/bmj/351/bmj.h4320.full.pdf

[82] Ashar YK, Sun M, Knight K, Flood TF, Anderson Z, Kaptchuk TJ, Wager TD. Open-Label Placebo Injection for Chronic Back Pain With Functional Neuroimaging: A Randomized Clinical Trial. JAMA Netw Open. 2024 Sep 3;7(9):e2432427. doi: 10.1001/jamanetworkopen.2024.32427. PMID: 39259542; PMCID: PMC11391328.

[83] Schaefer M, Kühnel A, Enge S. Open-label placebos reduce weight in obesity: a randomized controlled trial. Sci Rep. 2024 Sep 12;14(1):21311. doi: 10.1038/s41598-024-69866-7. PMID: 39266589; PMCID: PMC11392943.

[84] Park LC, Covi I. Non-blind placebo trial: an exploration of neurotic patients' responses to placebo when its inert content is disclosed. Arch Gen Psychiatry. 1965 Apr;12:36-45. PMID: 14258363.

[85] Masson J, McCarthy S. When elephants weep. London. Vintage. 1996. Preface

[86] Wartolowska K et al. Use of placebo controls in the evaluation of surgery: systematic review BMJ 2014;348:g3253

[87] McMillan FD. The placebo effect in animals. JAVMA 1999, 215: 7, 992-9

[88] Presumably as opposed to matching or other methods of comparison.

[89] Ivan Pavlov, 1849-1936. Pioneering and largely pre-Soviet psychologist who studied conditioned responses. Had crucial role in development of behavioural concepts.

[90] His death was so sudden and unexpected that some conspiracy theorists alleged a KGB plot.

[91] Gaynor J. et al. Effect of Perioperative Oral Carprofen on Postoperative Pain in Dogs Undergoing Surgery for Stabilization of Ruptured Cranial Cruciate Ligaments. Vet Ther. 2002 Winter;3(4):425-34.

[92] Curie A, Yang K, Kirsch I, Gollub RL, des Portes V, Kaptchuk TJ, Jensen KB. Placebo Responses in Genetically Determined Intellectual Disability: A Meta-Analysis. PLoS One. 2015 Jul 30;10(7):e0133316. doi: 10.1371/journal.pone.0133316. eCollection 2015.

[93] Grelotti J, Kaptchuk T. Placebo by proxy BMJ 2011; 343:d4345 doi: 10.1136/bmj.d4345

[94] http://www.bbc.co.uk/news/world-asia-china-42477083

[95] I realise that the word 'Oriental' makes some language Leninists uncomfortable but I am deliberately using it here for its old and often quite positive connotations of exoticism.

[96] Even in 1965, the mighty P&O shipping company expected me to use a single 10ml syringe to give ten crew members 1ml each of cholera vaccine, though I was allowed to use a fresh needle for each of them.

[97] Bishop F, Jacobsen E, Shaw J, Kaptchuk T. Participants' Experiences of Being Debriefed to Placebo Allocation in a Clinical Trial. Qual Health Res. 2012 Aug; 22(8): 1138–1149.

[98] Kaptchuk TJ, Kelley JM, Conboy LA, Davis RB, Kerr CE, Jacobson EE, Lembo AJ. Components of placebo effect: randomised controlled trial in patients with irritable bowel syndrome. British Medical Journal. 2008;336:999–1003.

[99] Interview with Kaptchuk for The Harvard Magazine Jan-Feb 2013

[100] Kaptchuk T, Miller F. Placebo Effects in Medicine N Engl J Med 2015; 373:8-9J: 10.1056/NEJMp1504023

[101] Dos Santos Maciel LY, Dos Santos Leite PM, Neto M, Mendonça AC, de Araujo CC, da Hora Santos Souza J, DeSantana JM. Comparison of the placebo effect between different non-penetrating acupuncture devices and real acupuncture in healthy subjects: a randomized clinical trial. BMC Complement Altern Med. 2016 Dec 15;16(1):518.

[102] Lowe C, Aiken A, Day AG, Depew W, Vanner SJ. Sham acupuncture is as efficacious as true acupuncture for the treatment of IBS: A randomized placebo controlled trial. Neurogastroenterol Motil. 2017 Jul;29(7). doi: 10.1111/nmo.13040. Epub 2017 Mar 2.

[103] Beevor, A. Berlin: the downfall 1945. London. Viking/Penguin 2002., p 212

[104] Sosis R. Psalms for Safety: Magico-Religious Responses to Threats of Terror. Curr Anthropol. 2007, 48; (6),903-11

[105] Jones RV. Most Secret War: British scientific intelligence 1939-1945. London, Coronet 1979. 275-7

[106] Ibid. p 492

[107] Ibid p 493

[108] In fact, the whole myth of dowsing, for water or lost items, is a tribute to the enduring power of the placebo effect. See: Testing Dowsing: The Failure of the Munich Experiments, J. T. Enright, Skeptical Inquirer, Volume 23, No. 1, January / February 1999

[109] en.wikipedia.org/wiki/ADE_651

[110] http://www.nachi.org/ultrasonic-pest-repellers.htm?loadbetadesign=0 accessed 21 Nov 2015

[111] https://www.theguardian.com/environment/2021/feb/06/weatherwatch-discredited-but-still-popular-enthusiasts-keep-faith-in-hail-cannon

[112] North, Adrian C. 2012. The effect of background music on the taste of wine. British Journal of Psychology. 103 (3): pp. 293-301.

[113] Cupping popular with Olympic athletes BBC report http://www.bbc.co.uk/news/health-37009240 accessed 8 Aug 2016.

[114] https://www.theguardian.com/commentisfree/2016/mar/26/after-brussels-attacks-develop-coping-strategy

[115] http://www.butterfliesandwheels.org/2010/why-having-chronic-illness-hasnt-turned-me-to-god/

[116] Krakauer J. Into the wild. New York Doubleday. 1997, 60

[117] Ehrenreich B. Smile or Die. How positive thinking fooled America and the world. London. Granta 2010.

[118] Gawande A. The power of negative thinking. New York Times. May 1st 2007.

[119] Lerner M The Belief in a Just World: A Fundamental Delusion. Plenum: New York. 1980

[120] Brown NJ, Sokal AD, Friedman HL. The complex dynamics of wishful thinking: The critical positivity ratio. Am Psychol. 2013 Dec;68(9):801-13

[121] Sokal A. Beyond the hoax. Oxford. OUP 2008.

[122] Weinberger E. What I Heard about Iraq. London Review of BooksVol. 27 No. 3 · 3 February 2005. Vol. 27.3-11

[123] Williams G. The age of agony. Chicago. Academy. 1975.

[124] de Botton A. A Point of View: The advantages of pessimism. BBC Radio 4 broadcast 12 Aug 2011. http://www.bbc.co.uk/news/magazine-14506129

[125] John Gray interviewed by Laurie Taylor. Going nowhere. Progress is an illusion and liberal humanists are adolescent romantics. New Humanist. Jan 11, 2006

[126] Cited in: http://new.spectator.co.uk/2015/10/fear-loneliness-and-nostalgia-a-return-to-johannesburg/ Justin Cartwright.

[127] Sundin J, Jones N, Greenberg N, et al. Mental health among commando, airborne and other UK infantry personnel. Occup Med (2010) 60 (7): 552-559.

[128] de Paula Couto, M. C. P., Weiss, D., Casper, M., & Rothermund, K. Contrasting paths to longevity: How personal and generalized views on aging differentially predict mortality. Psychology and Aging, 2025, 40(6), 583–593. https://doi.org/10.1037/pag0000902

[129] Başoğlu M1, Mineka S, Paker M, Aker T, Livanou M, Gök S. Psychological preparedness for trauma as a protective factor in survivors of torture. Psychol Med. 1997 Nov;27(6):1421-33.

[130] Essar N1, Palgi Y, Saar R, Ben-Ezra M.Pre-Traumatic Vaccination Intervention: can dissociative symptoms be reduced? Prehosp Disaster Med. 2010 May-Jun;25(3):278-84.

[131] Scheffer S. Death and the afterlife. Oxford. OUP. 2013 Reviewed in London Review of Books, Sept 25th 2014.

[132] The full title was: Candide, ou l'Optimisme.

[133] Thomson, N. Priming social affiliation promotes morality – Regardless of religion. Personal Individ Diff, 2015. 75, 195-200 DOI: 10.1016/j.paid.2014.11.022

[134] https://yougov.co.uk/news/2016/03/26/o-we-of-little-faith/

[135] Hitchens P. The rage against God. London, Bloomsbury, 2010. 75

[136] http://hitchensblog.mailonsunday.co.uk/2008/02/is-the-church-o.html

[137] Berry, M. Post-Atheism: A Mechanist's Journey from Christian Materialism to Material Spirituality. 2001 ISBN-10: 0759674574

[138] Furnham A. Horne G. Who Beliefs[sic] in Alternative Medicine?. Health, 2024, 16, 1235-1241. doi: 10.4236/health.2024.1612085.

[139] Vinar O. Dependence on a placebo; a case report. Brit J Psychiat. 1969, 115; 189-90

[140] d'Holbach, Baron The system of Nature (Trans S Wilkinson) London. 1820. NB The authorship is erroneously attributed to Mirebaud.

[141] Wink P1, Scott J. Does religiousness buffer against the fear of death and dying in late adulthood? Findings from a longitudinal study. J Gerontol B Psychol Sci Soc Sci. 2005 Jul;60(4):P207-14.

[142] Jong J, Ross R, Philip T, et al. The religious correlates of death anxiety: a systematic review and meta-analysis Relig Brain Behav. doi.org/10.1080/2153599X.2016.1238844

[143] Kors, A C. Atheism in France 1650-1729. Vol 1: the orthodox sources of disbelief. Princeton, 1990. p 28

[144] http://www.cell.com/current-biology/pdf/S0960-9822%2815%2901167-7.pdf Decety et al. access ed 19 Nov 2015

[145] http://www.pbs.org/wnet/religionandethics/2015/02/20/february-20-2015-rabbi-jonathan-sacks-science-religion/25268/

[146] Hood, R., Spilka, B., Hunsberger, B., Gorsuch, R. The psychology of religion: An empirical approach (second edition), New York: Guilford. 1996, 103-104).

[147] Solomon S, Greenberg J, Pyszczynski T. The worm at the core: on the role of death in life. London, Penguin. 2015.

[148] Jensen K, Kirsch I, Odmalm S, Kaptchuk T, Ingvarb M. Classical conditioning of analgesic and hyperalgesic pain responses without conscious awareness Proc Natl Acad Sci U S A. 2015 Jun 23; 112(25): 7863–7867.

[149] I only recall dealing with (or hearing immediate colleagues discuss) one case in two decades of acute medicine and psychiatry and he was discovered unexpectedly.

[150] Curlin FA, Lantos JD, Roach CJ, Sellergren SA, Chin MH. Religious Characteristics of U.S. Physicians: A National Survey. Journal of General Internal Medicine. 2005;20(7):629-634. doi:10.1111/j.1525-1497.2005.0119.x.

[151] "Weaver J. Sorrows of a century: interpreting suicide in New Zealand 1900–2000. Montreal, McGill–Queens, 2014."

[152] Chivers T. https://www.buzzfeed.com/tomchivers/how-doctors-want-to-die?utm_term=.edBVgYdYV#.dpp8Xxex8

[153] Williams N, Dunford C, Knowles A, Warner J. Public attitudes to life-sustaining treatments and euthanasia in dementia. . 2007 Dec;22(12):1229-34.

[154] Van Wijmen M, Pasman H, Widdershoven G, Onwuteaka- Philipsen B. Continuing or forgoing treatment at the end of life? Preferences of the general public and people with an advance directive. J.Med.Ethics. Published online September 2nd 2014. 10.1136/medethics-2013-101544

[155] Note for non-Londoners: Cadogan Square is still a very up-market address.

[156] Rev H A Wilson in (N Longmate, Ed) The Home Front. An anthology 1938-45. London, Chatto and Windus, 1981. 79-80.

[157] American Evangelicals like Billy Graham "have no doubt that God does intervene on occasion to heal people without the aid of medicine " but He heals them without the need for saints or relics. https://billygraham.org/answer/does-god-still-heal-people-like-he-did-when-jesus-was-on-earth-if-he-does-then-why-do-we-need-doctors-and-medicine-shouldnt-a-strong-faith-be-enough-and-isnt-that-what-god-wants-us-to-have/

[158] Grou JN (Trans. Dalby J) How to pray. London. James Clarke. 1964, 71.

158 John Dominic Crossan; Richard G. Watts (1999). Who is Jesus?: answers to your questions about the historical Jesus. Westminster. John Knox Press. p. 64. ISBN 978-0-664-25842-9.

[160] www.whywontgodhealamputees.com/

[161] http://www.ncregister.com/blog/benjamin-wiker/st.-teresa-of-calcutta-pray-for-stephen-hawking

[162] Duffin, J. The Doctor Was Surprised; or, How to Diagnose a Miracle. Bulletin of the History of Medicine, 2007: 81 (4) 699-729

[163] Duffin J. Medical miracles: doctors, saints and healing in the modern world. Oxford University Press. 2009.

[164] Cornwell J. The pope in winter. London, Penguin. 2005, 106.

[165] Rees W, Dover S, Low-Beer T, "Patients with terminal cancer" who have neither terminal illness nor cancer. Brit Med J. 1987, 295;318-9

[166] Trof RJ, Beishuizen A, Wondergem MJ, Strack van Schijndel RJ. Spontaneous remission of acute myeloid leukaemia after recovery from sepsis. Neth J Med. 2007 Jul-Aug;65(7):259-62.

[167] Ifrah N, James JM, Viguie F, Marie JP, Zittoun R. Spontaneous remission in adult acute leukemia. Cancer. 1985 Sep 1;56(5):1187-90.

[168] Lachant NA, Goldberg J, Nelson DA, Gottlieb AJ Spontaneous remission in acute myelogenous leukemia in the adult. Am J Med. 1979 Oct;67(4):687-92.

[169] Keefer MJ, Weber MJ, Bottomley SS, Solanki DL, Hosty TA Peripheral blood remission of hairy cell leukemia after transfusion hepatitis. Am J Hematol. 1987 Jul;25(3):277-84.

[170] Lokich J. Spontaneous regression of metastatic renal cancer. Case report and literature review. Am J Clin Oncol. 1997 Aug;20(4):416-8.

[171] Dussan C, Zubor P, Fernandez M, Yabar A, Szunyogh N, Visnovsky J. Spontaneous regression of a breast carcinoma: a case report. Gynecol Obstet Invest. 2008;65(3):206-11

[172] Buckman R, Sabbagh K. Magic or Medicine: an investigation into healing. London, Pan, 1993. 149.

[173] Cornwell J. The pope in winter. London, Penguin. 2005, 89.

[174] Nine years later, he was killed by a projectile that went straight through his head.

[175] Brewer C. Homicide during a psychomotor seizure. Medical Journal of Australia. 1971; 1: 857-9

[176] Kuzmanovski I, Cvetkovska E, Babunovska M, Kiteva Trencevska G, Kuzmanovska B, Boshkovski B, Isjanovska R. Seizure outcome following medical treatment of mesial temporal lobe epilepsy: Clinical phenotypes and prognostic factors. Clin Neurol Neurosurg. 2016 May;144:91-5. doi: 10.1016/j.clineuro.2016.03.018. Epub 2016 Mar 24. PMID: 27037863.

[177] Benson H, Dusek JA, Sherwood JB, et al. Study of the Therapeutic Effects of Intercessory Prayer (STEP) in cardiac bypass patients: a multicenter randomized trial of uncertainty and certainty of receiving intercessory prayer. Am Heart J. 2006 Apr;151(4):934-42.

[178] Review by Gavin Francis of Spinney L. Pale Rider: The Spanish Flu of 1918 and How It Changed the World. Lond Rev Books. 40(2) 25 Jan 2018, 3-6

[179] Drescher E. Quitting Religion, But Not the Practice of Prayer http://www.religiondispatches.org/archive/atheologies/6973/ accessed 27 March 2013.

[180] Cha KY, Wirth DP, Lobo RA. Does prayer influence the success of in vitro fertilization-embryo transfer? Journal of Reproductive Medicine 46:781-787

[181] http://www.quackwatch.org/11Ind/wirthstudy.html

[182] Gaudia G. About Intercessory Prayer. www.butterfliesandwheels.com/articleprint.php?num=282 Accessed 16 Aug 2011

[183] Roberts L, Ahmed I, Hall S, Davison A. Intercessory prayer for the alleviation of ill health. Cochrane Database Syst Rev. 2009 Apr 15;(2):CD000368.

[184] Sarzeaud, N. A New Document on the Appearance of the Shroud of Turin from Nicole Oresme: Fighting False Relics and False Rumours in the Fourteenth Century. Journal of Medieval History, 2025. 1–18. doi.org/10.1080/03044181.2025.2546884

[185] http://www.bbc.co.uk/news/uk-northern-ireland-18476310

[186] Ireland has recently moved from 25th to 17th place. 12

[187] Nuzzi G. (Trans: F. Moore) Merchants in the Temple: inside Pope Francis's secret battle against corruption in the Vatican. New York. Macmillan. 2015. Ch. 2 The Saint's Factory.

[188] https://www.scottishlegal.com/articles/and-finally-doctored-records

[189] https://rjosephhoffmann.wordpress.com/2009/12/28/religion-2010-wish-list/

[190] Kaptchuk T, Kerr C, Zanger A Placebo Controls, Exorcisms and the Devil, Lancet. 2009 Oct 10; 374(9697): 1234.

[191] Hill C. The world turned upside down. Radical ideas during the English revolution London. Pelican 1975, 87

[192] Book of Kings 1, v 18

[193] Kaptchuk T, Miller F. Placebo Effects in Medicine N Engl J Med 2015; 373:8-9J: 10.1056/NEJMp1504023

[194] Kerr D, Davidson S. Gastrointestinal intolerance to oral iron preparations. Lancet 1958. 2:489-92.

[195] Kam-Hansen S. et al Altered placebo and drug labeling changes the outcome of episodic migraine attacks. Sci Transl Med. 2014 Jan 8;6(218):218ra5. doi: 10.1126/scitranslmed.3006175.

[196] Rubin GJ, Nieto-Hernandez R, Wessely S. Idiopathic environmental intolerance attributed to electromagnetic fields (formerly 'electromagnetic hypersensitivity'): An updated systematic review of provocation studies. Bioelectromagnetics. 2010 Jan;31(1):1-11. doi: 10.1002/bem.20536. PMID: 19681059.

[197] Rubin GJ, Hillert L, Nieto-Hernandez R, van Rongen E, Oftedal G. Do people with idiopathic environmental intolerance attributed to electromagnetic fields display physiological effects when exposed to electromagnetic fields? A systematic review of provocation studies. Bioelectromagnetics. 2011 Dec;32(8):593-609. doi: 10.1002/bem.20690.

[198] Rubin GJ, Burns M, Wessely S. Possible psychological mechanisms for "wind turbine syndrome". On the windmills of your mind. Noise Health. 2014 Mar-Apr;16(69):116-22

[199] Owen RD. The Convulsionists of Saint-Medard The Atlantic Monthly. February-March, 1864 Online at http://www.romancatholicism.org/jansenism/convulsionists.htm accessed 12 Jan 2013.

[200] Taibbi M.The Great Derangement. New York. Spiegel & Grau, 2008

[201] Showalter E. Hystories. Hysterical Epidemics and Modern Media. New York, Columbia, 1998. 27

[202] 'Off label' means prescribing a drug to treat a condition for which it has not been specifically licensed and that does not appear on the information sheet or 'label'.

[203] Ali R, Thomas P, White J, McGregor C, Danz C, Gowing L, Stegink A, Athanasos P. Antagonist-precipitated heroin withdrawal under anaesthetic prior to maintenance naltrexone treatment: determinants of withdrawal severity. Drug Alc Rev. 2003 Dec;22(4):425-31.

[204] Bell JR, Young MR, Masterman SC, Morris A, Mattick RP, Bammer G. A pilot study of naltrexone-accelerated detoxifcation in opioid dependence.Med J Aust 1999;171:26-30

[205] Brewer C. [Octreotide in rapid opiate detoxification.] La octreotida en la desintoxicacion rapida de opiaceos. Rev Espan Drogodepend 1999;24:426-7

[206] Bertelli G. Di Bella treatment was worthless. www.quackwatch.org/01QuackeryRelatedTopics/Cancer/dibella.html

[207] Italian Study Group for the Di Bella Multitherapy Trials. Evaluation of an unconventional cancer treatment (the Di Bella multitherapy): results of phase II trials in Italy. BMJ 1999; 318 : 224

[208] https://www.welt.de/gesundheit/plus254695428/Globuli-statt-Antibiotika-Warum-eine-Studie-zum-Vergleich-der-Wirksamkeit-jetzt-abgebrochen-wurde.html?icid=search.product.onsitesearch

[209] Vickers A et al. Do certain countries produce only positive results? A systematic review of controlled trials. Controlled Clinical Trials 1998:19(2);159-66

[210] Editorial. China's medical research integrity questioned. Lancet, 2015.385;9976,1365

[211] Ahn AC, et al. Electrical properties of acupuncture points and meridians: a systematic review. Bioelectromagnetics. 2008 May;29(4):245-56. doi: 10.1002/bem.20403.

[212] Berson EL1, Remulla JF, Rosner B, Sandberg MA, Weigel-DiFranco C. Evaluation of patients with retinitis pigmentosa receiving electric stimulation, ozonated blood, and ocular surgery in Cuba. Arch Ophthalmol. 1996 May;114(5):560-3.

[213] Trofim Lysenko (1898-1976) was Stalin's favourite agronomist. His ideologically-driven genetic theories damaged food production and some of his opponents disappeared into the gulags.

[214] Isaacson W. Steve Jobs: the exclusive biography. London. Bloomsbury 2012.

[215] By Kunzli, Naude and Pendleton, London. Orion. 2003

[216] http://drsheelasuresh.wordpress.com/2007/01/25/lecture-18-chronic-diseases-psora/ accessed 20 Mar 2013

[217] http://www.helium.com/items/1887921-the-concept-of-psora-in-homeopathic-medicine accessed 21 Mar 2013

[218] http://www.homeoint.org/morrell/articles/pm_miasm.htm accessed 21 Mar 2013

[219] I once treated a teenaged girl who had taken a large dose of quinine as an abortifacient before the 1967 Abortion Act made such desperate but common expedients unnecessary. She became blind – fortunately, not permanently – but not feverish. Her foetus was spared the same fate because she did actually abort.

[220] http://www.angelfire.com/mb2/quinine/allergy.html Accessed.

[221] http://www.catholicculture.org/culture/library/view.cfm?recnum=1340

[222] Congregation for Doctrine of the Faith Prot. 89/78-174 98 July 24, 2003

[223] Father Edward McNamara, professor of liturgy at the Regina Apostolorum Pontifical University. ZENIT Rome, 14 Sept. 2004

[224] Bell IR, Brooks AJ, Howerter A, Jackson N, Schwartz GE. Short-term effects of repeated olfactory administration of homeopathic sulphur or pulsatilla on electroencephalographic alpha power in healthy young adults. Homeopathy. 2011 Oct;100(4):203-11.

[225] http://www.parliamentlive.tv/Event/Index/7374b758-5e81-430e-8f7b-13d43ec13b9a

[226] Chapman G. Rapid Response to: Torjesen I. Civil servants suppress evidence on homeopathy on NHS website after lobbying from prince's charity. BMJ 2013;346:f1071

[227] Blackie. Margery G. The challenge of homoeopathy: the patient, not the cure. London : Macdonald and Jane's, 1975.

[228] http://www.britishhomeopathic.org/bha-charity/how-we-can-help/medicine-a-z/a-closer-look-at-pulsatilla/

[229] Scrofula - a disfiguring and now rare tuberculous skin disease.

[230] When my own private dermatologist was appointed to the Queen's medical household, his waiting list quickly became so long that I reluctantly took my epidermis elsewhere.

[231] Robb G. The discovery of France. London. Picador 2008 p 132

[232] Williams NA, Lee MG, Hanchard B, Barrow KO. Hepatic cirrhosis in Jamaica. West Indian Med J. 1997 Jun;46(2):60-2.

[233] Likhitsup A, Chen VL, Fontana RJ. Estimated Exposure to 6 Potentially Hepatotoxic Botanicals in US Adults. JAMA Netw Open. 2024 Aug

1;7(8):e2425822. doi: 10.1001/jamanetworkopen.2024.25822. PMID: 39102266; PMCID: PMC11301549.

[234] Loftfield E, O'Connell CP, Abnet CC, et al. Multivitamin Use and Mortality Risk in 3 Prospective US Cohorts. JAMA Netw Open. 2024;7(6):e2418729.doi:10.1001/jamanetworkopen.2024.18729

[235] Tessier A, Cortese M, Yuan C, et al. Consumption of Olive Oil and Diet Quality and Risk of Dementia-Related Death. JAMA Netw Open. 2024;7(5):e2410021. doi:10.1001/jamanetworkopen.2024.10021

[236] Culpeper N. Complete Herbal. Ware. Wordsworth. 1995. 271

[237] Kipling's verse. Inclusive edition 1885-1926 London. Hodder 1929. p 547

[238] Jørgensen CH, Pedersen B, Tønnesen H. The efficacy of disulfiram for the treatment of alcohol use disorder. Alcohol Clin Exp Res. 2011 Oct;35(10):1749-58

[239] Berglund M, Thelander S, Salaspuro M, Franck J, Andréasson S, Öjehagen A. Treatment of Alcohol Abuse: An Evidence-Based Review. Alcoholism: Clinical and Experimental Research, 27:1645-1656, 2003)

[240] Skinner MD, Lahmek P, Pham H, Aubin HJ . Disulfiram efficacy in the treatment of alcohol dependence: a meta-analysis. PLoS One. 2014 Feb 10;9(2):e87366.

[241] Brewer C, Streel E, Skinner M. Supervised disulfiram's superior effectiveness in alcoholism treatment: ethical, methodological and psychological aspects. Alc. Alcohol. 2017,1-7

[242] Lobmaier PP1, Kunøe N, Gossop M, Waal H. Naltrexone depot formulations for opioid and alcohol dependence: a systematic review. CNS Neurosci Ther. 2011 Dec;17(6):629-36. doi: 10.1111/j.1755-5949.2010.00194.x.

[243] Opheim A, Benth JŠ, Solli KK, Kloster PS, Fadnes LT, Kunøe N, Gaulen Z, Tanum L. Risk of relapse to non-opioid addictive substances among opioid dependent patients treated with an opioid receptor antagonist or a partial agonist: A randomized clinical trial. Contemp Clin Trials. 2023 Dec;135:107360. doi: 10.1016/j.cct.2023.107360. Epub 2023 Oct 19. PMID: 37865138.

[244] Opheim A, Gaulen Z, Solli KK, Latif ZE, Fadnes LT, Benth JŠ, Kunøe N, Tanum L. Risk of Relapse Among Opioid-Dependent Patients Treated With Extended-Release Naltrexone or Buprenorphine-Naloxone: A Randomized Clinical Trial. Am J Addict. 2021 Sep;30(5):453-460. doi: 10.1111/ajad.13151. PMID: 34487395.

[245] Ernst E. A scientist in wonderland: a memoir of searching for truth and finding trouble. Exeter, Imprint. 2015.

[246] Park R. Voodoo Science: The road from foolishness to fraud. New York. OUP. 2000. 65 (Cited by Barker Bausell. Snake Oil Science. Op cit.)

[247] The relevant verses are 4:157-8 A widely-read modern critique by the S African Muslim preacher Ahmed Deedat is titled 'Crucifixion or Cruci-fiction?'.

[248] http://www.cfnews.org/page88/files/2191f0efb39c5c77282dd8313862eb87-307.html

[249] Hedges C. War is a force that gives us meaning. New York, Anchor 2003. 43

[250] Storr A. Feet of Clay: a study of gurus. London. Harper Collins.1996. Ch 6.

[251] The schisms persist. In September 2016, Pope Francis preached in a near empty stadium during a visit to Tbilisi, Georgia after the dominant Orthodox church insisted that "As long as there are dogmatic differences between our churches, Orthodox believers will not participate in their prayers". An Orthodox priest said: "Can you imagine how it would be if a Sunni preacher came to Shia Iran and conducted prayers in a stadium or somewhere else? Such a thing could not be." www.bbc.co.uk/news/world-europe-37530407

[252] Phillips A. Becoming Freud: the making of a psychoanalyst. New Haven. Yale. 25-6.

[253] Masson JM. Final Analysis, op. cit. 182.

[254] Ehrman B. Misquoting Jesus: the story behind who changed the bible and why. San Francisco. Harper. 2005 passim.

[255] Ehrman B. Forged: Writing in the Name of God—Why the Bible's Authors Are Not Who We Think They Are. HarperCollins, USA. 2011. passim

[256] Holland T. In the shadow of the sword: the battle for global empire and the end of the ancient world. London. Little Brown. 2012. 190

[257] Ibid, 44

[258] Masson JM. Final Analysis. op. cit. 183

[259] Ibid. 129

[260] Cioffi F. Book review . New Society. 29 Nov 1979. p503.

[261] Masson JM. Final Analysis, op cit. 209

[262] Storr A. Feet of clay. A study of gurus. London. Harper Collins. 2013.

[263] Witkowski T, Zatonski M. Psychology gone wrong. Boca Raton. Brown Walker 2015.

[264] They fuck you up, your mum and dad… 'This be the verse' Collected Poems Farrar Straus and Giroux, 2001.

[265] Masson J. Final analysis : the making and unmaking of a psychoanalyst London. Harper Collins, 1991. 206\

[266] Masson JM. My Father's Guru. New York, Ballantine. 2003, xi

[267] Ibid. 152-3

[268] Bosworth R, Sins of the Sisters, reviewing Wolf H. (trans. R. Martin) The Nuns of Sant 'Ambrogio: The True story of a Convent Scandal. Literary Review. 2015. 428. Feb. 32-3

[269] I met and interviewed him after the original draft of this chapter. He seems a very happy man now.

[270] Masson JM. Final Analysis, op cit. 8-9.

[271] Ibid. 153

[272] Masson J. Final Analysis p 172

[273] Masson JM. (Transl. and Ed.) The complete letters of Sigmund Freud to Wilhelm Fliess. Cambridge, Mass. Belknap/Harvard. 1985.

[274] Glaser F. Interview. Addiction 2001, 96.1710.

[275] Masson http://www.theatlantic.com/magazine/archive/1984/02/freud-and-the-seduction-theory/376313/

[276] Masson J. The Assault on Truth: Freud's suppression of the seduction theory. Toronto, Collins. 1984. 99

[277] Obholzer K. The Wolf-Man sixty years later. Conversations with Freud's patient. London. Routledge. 1982. Passim

[278] Torrey EF. Ezra Pound: The roots of treason. London. Sidgwick and Jackson. 1984.

[279] Obholzer K. (Trans. M. Shaw) The wolf-man sixty years later. Conversations with Freud's patient. London. Routledge. 1982.

[280] http://www2.webster.edu/~woolflm/brunswick.html

[281] Anon. Fees for medical examination for insurance. BMJ.Sept 3rd 1910, 662-3.

[282] I haven't gone through it myself but a friend who possesses every volume, spread over many yards of her bookshelves, confirmed its absence.

[283] James 1st/6th A counterblaste to tobacco. 1604 http://www.laits.utexas.edu/poltheory/james/blaste/blaste.html accessed 23 Feb 2012

[284] DeSteno D. How God Works. The science behind the benefits of religion. New York, Simon and Schuster 127-34

[285] Dawkins R. The God Delusion. 167

[286] Hitchens C. The portable atheist. Philadelphia. Da Capo/Perseus. 2007.

[287] An American book with a promising title - Kuby L. Faith and the placebo effect. An argument for self-healing. Novato CA. Origin Press. 2001 - turned out to be an uncritical endorsement of faith healing and how it cured the author's breast cancer. It hardly discusses alternative explanations for her 'cure' and doesn't look at the wider issue.

[288] Joyce C. Is god a placebo? Forsch Komplementärmed 1998 (5) Suool 1, 47-51.

[289] Lobdell W. Losing my religion. How I lost my faith reporting on religion in America – and found unexpected peace. New York. Collins. 2009

[290] It may also explain why only 17 papers come up after a search for 'god AND placebo' on PubMed. In 11 of those, 'god' turns out to be either a reference to studies of the Thunder-God vine, tripterygium hypoglaucum (a Chinese herb with possible contraceptive effects) or to the fact that one of the authors works at a hospital named after St John of God.

[291] cited in Burleigh M. Earthly Powers. Ch 1

[292] Dennett D. Breaking the Spell; religion as a natural phenomenon. London, Penguin, 2007. 137

[293] Thomson JA, Aukofer C. Why we believe in god(s). A concise guide to the science of faith. Charlottesville. Pitchstone. 2011

[294] Wathey JC. The Illusion of God's Presence: the biological origins of spiritual longing. Amherst NY. Prometheus. 2016

[295] Kapuscinski R. Shah of Shahs. London, Penguin, 2006. 130

[296] Ferguson N. The ascent of money. London. Penguin. 2009. 392

[297] Brewer C. Murder and the McNaghten Rules: the importance of adequate medical investigation. Australia and New Zealand Journal of Criminology. 1971;4:94-100

[298] Trimble M. The soul in the brain: the cerebral basis of language, art and belief. Baltimore, Johns Hopkins. 2007. Passim

[299] Aziz H. Did Prophet Mohammad (PBUH) have epilepsy? A neurological analysis, Epilepsy Behav,103,A, 2020, doi.org/10.1016/j.yebeh.2019.106654.

[300] Carrazana E, DeToledo J, Tatum W et al. Epilepsy and religious experiences: Voodoo possession. Epilepsia. 1999. 40(2) 239-41

[301] Yaden, D. B., Eichstaedt, J. C., Schwartz, H. A., Kern, M. L., Le Nguyen, K. D., Wintering, N. A., Hood, R. W., Jr., & Newberg, AB The language of ineffability: Linguistic analysis of mystical experiences. Psychology of Religion and Spirituality 2016. 8(3), 244–252. https://doi.org/10.1037/rel0000043

[302] Persinger MA The temporal lobe: the biological basis of the god experience. In: (Joseph R. Ed) Neurotheology. Brain, science, spirituality, religious experience. San Jose. University Press. 2003. 273.

[303] Linden S C, Harris M, Whitaker C, Healy D. Religion and psychosis: the effects of the Welsh religious revival in 1904–1905. Psychol Med (2010), 40, 1317–1323.

[304] Brewer C. Incidence of post-abortion psychosis: a prospective study. Br Med J. 1977 Feb 19;1(6059):476-7. doi: 10.1136/bmj.1.6059.476. PMID: 837169; PMCID: PMC1605106.

[305] Macalpine, Ida and Hunter, Richard 'The Insanity of King George III: A Classic Case of Porphyria'. Brit Med J.1966; 1; 65-71

[306] Macalpine I, Hunter R, Rimington C (January 1968). "Porphyria in the royal houses of Stuart, Hanover, and Prussia. A follow-up study of George 3d's illness". Br Med J 1 (5583): 7–18.

[307] www.nytimes.com/1981/08/16/arts/rimsky-korsakov-s-mozart-and-salieri.html

[308] Peters T, Wilkinson D. King George III and porphyria: a clinical re-examination of the historical evidence History of Psychiatry 2010. 21(1) 3–19

[309] Peters T. King George III and the porphyria myth – causes, consequences and re-evaluation of his mental illness with computer diagnostics. Clin Med 2015 Vol 15, No 2: 168–72

[310] Lithium is one of Australia's few useful contributions to psychiatry, as opposed to its impressive efforts in other medical fields. In the 1950s, Dr Frank Cade gave lithium salts to rats to study their effects on heart function and noticed that the rats became less active. On this rather crude basis, they were given to over-active, manic patients and seemed to be helpful, as was later confirmed in RCTs. Some early patients died from excessive lithium doses before it became easy to measure its level in the blood. This is why new treatments need to be tested for both good and bad effects. Nobody knew then how lithium worked and it is still not clear but that doesn't necessarily matter provided we know that a) it really does work better than placebo medication and that b) the bad effects don't outweigh the good ones.

[311] Peters T. et al The nature of King James VI/I's medical conditions: new approaches to the diagnosis. History of Psychiatry 2012. 23(3) 277–290

[312] Bagley C. The evaluation of a suicide prevention scheme by an ecological method. Soc Sci Med. 1968 Mar;2(1):1-14.

[313] Jones, D. Self-poisoning with drugs: the past twenty years in Sheffield. Brit. Med.J. 1977; 1,28-9.

[314] Brewer C, Farmer R. Self poisoning in 1984: a prediction that didn't come true. Brit. Med. J. 1985;290:391

[315] Barraclough BM, Jennings C. Suicide prevention by the Samaritans. A controlled study of effectiveness. Lancet. 1977 Jul 30;2(8031):237-9.

[316] Gibbons JS, Butler J, Urwin P, Gibbons JL. Evaluation of a social work service for self-poisoning patients. Br J Psychiatry. 1978 Aug;133:111-8.

[317] Letter to Keats' brother and sister, Spring 1819, kept by Robert Kennedy (assassinated 1967) in his desk drawer.

[318] A bronze statue of Servetus in the nearby French town of Annemasse was melted down by the Vichy government in 1942 because Servetus stood for freedom of conscience. It was re-cast and restored in 1960.

[319] Buckley GT Atheism in the English Renaissance. NY, Russell and Russell.1965. p24

[320] Bickerton TH. A Medical history of Liverpool from the earliest days to the year 1920. 1936. London. John Murray. p213

[321] http://recoveredhistories.org/paemphlet1.php?catid=59

[322] Wootton D New Histories of Atheism In: Hunter M and Wootton D Eds. Atheism from the reformation to the enlightenment. Oxford. Clarendon, 1992

[323] Seamus Berry in London Review of Books 25 Feb 2010, reviewing Anna Letitia Barbauld: voice of the enlightenment by William McCarthy Johns Hopkins. 2008.

[324] Shepherd JA. A history of the Liverpool Medical Institution . Liverpool LMI 1979

[325] Benedetti F. Placebo Effects (second edition). Oxford. OUP. 2014

[326] Edwards G, Orford J, Egert S, Guthrie S, Hawker A, Hensman C, Mitcheson E, Oppenheimer E, Taylor C. et al. Alcoholism: a controlled trial of 'treatment' and 'advice'. Quart J Stud Alc 1977;38:1004-33.

[328] Hróbjartsson A, Gøtzsche PC. Is the placebo powerless? An analysis of clinical trials comparing placebo with no treatment. N Engl J Med. 2001 May 24;344(21):1594-602. doi: 10.1056/NEJM200105243442106. Erratum in: N Engl J Med 2001 Jul 26;345(4):304. PMID: 11372012.

[329] Howick J, Friedemann C, Tsakok M, Watson R, Tsakok T, Thomas J, Perera R, Fleming S, Heneghan C. Are treatments more effective than placebos? A systematic review and meta-analysis. PLoS One. 2013 May 15;8(5):e62599. doi: 10.1371/journal.pone.0062599. Erratum in: PLoS One. 2016 Jan 15;11(1):e0147354. doi: 10.1371/journal.pone.0147354. PMID: 23690944; PMCID: PMC3655171.

[330] Foddy B. Justifying deceptive placebos. In: (Eds. A Raz and C Harris) Placebo Talks. Oxford. OUP. 2016.52-68.

[331] Kaptchuk TJ et al. Placebos without Deception: A Randomized Controlled Trial in Irritable Bowel Syndrome PLoS One. 2010; 5(12): e15591.

[332] Druart L, Graham Longsworth SE, Terrisse H, Locher C, Blease C, Rolland C, Pinsault N. If only they knew! A non-inferiority randomized controlled trial comparing deceptive and open-label placebo in healthy individuals. Eur J Pain. 2024 Mar;28(3):491-501. doi: 10.1002/ejp.2204. Epub 2023 Nov 15. PMID: 37965922.

[333] Gerdesmeyer L, Klueter T, Rahlfs VW, Muderis MA, Saxena A, Gollwitzer H, Harrasser N, Stukenberg M, Prehn-Kristensen A. Randomized Placebo-Controlled Placebo Trial to Determine the Placebo Effect Size. Pain Physician. 2017 Jul;20(5):387-396. PMID: 28727701.

[334] Hardman D, Miller F. J Med Ethics Dec 2024. doi:10.1136/jme-2024-110270

[335] https://www.bbc.co.uk/news/health-45721670

[336] Moerman D. Looking at placebos through a cultural lens and finding meaning. In: (Eds. A Raz and C Harris) Placebo Talks. Oxford. OUP. 2016. 111.

[337] De Botton A. Religion for atheists. Op cit. 242.

[338] https://www.thetimes.com/uk/healthcare/article/king-charles-doctor-nhs-problems-homeopathy-708tfzp9b

[339] Pereira Gray DJ, Sidaway-Lee K, White E, Thorne A, Evans PH. Continuity of care with doctors-a matter of life and death? A systematic review of continuity of care and mortality. BMJ Open. 2018 Jun 28;8(6):e021161. doi: 10.1136/bmjopen-2017-021161

[340] Ernst E. A scientist in wonderland: a memoir of searching for truth and finding trouble. Exeter, Imprint. 2015.

[341] Ernst E. Charles, the Alternative King. An unauthorised biography. Societas. 2023.

[342] Brewer C. Dictators of medical fashion. General Practitioner. 1986. July 18th

[343] Gorski D. The rebranding of CAM as "harnessing the power of placebo" https://sciencebasedmedicine.org/the-rebranding-of-cam/

[344] Interview with Kaptchuk for The Harvard Magazine Jan-Feb 2013

[345] Or as Sir John Gielgud put it: "I'm an actor. Of course I can play a heterosexual!"

[346] Possible essay question for philosophy and bioethics students: 'AI counselling cannot be sincere. Discuss.'

[347] Wagner B, Horn A, Maercker A. Internet-based versus face-to-face cognitive-behavioral intervention for depression: A randomized controlled non-inferiority trial J Affect Disord, 2014, 152 , 113 – 121

[348] https://www.spectator.co.uk/article/its-time-to-make-friends-with-ai/

[349] http://www.bbc.co.uk/news/av/world-europe-40101661/robotic-reverend-blesses-worshippers-in-eight-languages

[350] Cupitt D. John Robinson and the language of faith in God. In: (Ed. Colin Slee) Honest to God 40 years on. London. SCM. 2004. 44

[351] Jefferson T. Notes on the State of Virginia. In: (Ed. Merrill Peterson) The portable Jefferson. London. Penguin 1977, 211.

[352] Text of the Treaty of Tripoli, 1797

Index